Experts' Perspectives on Medical Advances

This book series presents Chinese experts' perspectives on recent developments in clinical medicine. Written by leading Chinese experts in related fields, a wide variety of emerging and hot topics in internal medicine, surgery, oncology, neurosurgery, and ophthalmonology, etc., is covered by the series. Each title in this series covers a disease or a group of diseases, focusing on the basic knowledge, development and the latest research progress of clinical practice. This series is a practical and useful resource for researchers and practitioners in related subjects, as well as for general interest readers.

Jian-Guo Wen
Editor

Progress in Clean Intermittent Catheterization

科学技术文献出版社
SCIENTIFIC AND TECHNICAL DOCUMENTATION PRESS

Springer

Editor
Jian-Guo Wen
Pediatric Urodynamic Center/Department of Urology
First Affiliated Hospital of Zhengzhou University
Zhengzhou, China

ISSN 2948-1023 ISSN 2948-1031 (electronic)
Experts' Perspectives on Medical Advances
ISBN 978-981-97-5023-8 ISBN 978-981-97-5021-4 (eBook)
https://doi.org/10.1007/978-981-97-5021-4

The original submitted manuscript has been translated into English. The translation was done using artificial intelligence. A subsequent revision was performed by the author(s) to further refine the work and to ensure that the translation is appropriate concerning content and scientific correctness. It may, however, read stylistically different from a conventional translation.

Translation from the Chinese Simplified language edition: "清洁间歇性导尿术文建国2021观点" by Jian-Guo Wen, © Scientific and Technical Documentation Press 2021. Published by Scientific and Technical Documentation Press. All Rights Reserved.

Jointly published with Scientific and Technical Documentation Press
The print edition is not for sale in China (Mainland). Customers from China (Mainland) please order the print book from: Scientific and Technical Documentation Press.
Experts' Perspectives on Medical Advances

This Springer imprint is published by the registered company Springer Nature Singapore Pte Ltd.
The registered company address is: 152 Beach Road, #21-01/04 Gateway East, Singapore 189721, Singapore

Preface

Clean Intermittent Catheterization (CIC) is a method of regularly emptying the bladder through the urethra or bladder stoma using a catheter under clean conditions. It can prevent bladder overdistension, treat urinary incontinence, and prevent kidney damage. CIC is simple to operate and can be performed by the patient themselves or their family members in the community or at home.

In 1972, Lapides and others proposed CIC for the treatment of neurogenic bladder (NB), which quickly became a life-saving treatment for patients who could not empty their bladder autonomously. After more than 40 years of development, CIC has been recognized by the International Continence Society (ICS) as the preferred treatment method for bladder emptying. With the popularization of CIC, it effectively prevents vesicoureteral reflux (VUR) and kidney damage and reduces the rate of bladder augmentation in patients with NB. However, in many countries, the application of CIC is not yet widespread, and there are not many literature reports on CIC, especially in children. The European Urological Association has recommended that CIC can start in newborns with NB voiding difficulties. The CIC may accompany the patient's life, starting early and getting used to CIC early, which helps the patient integrate into society as soon as possible and reduce the occurrence of psychological problems. In order for patients or their families to master CIC, relevant training is very important. However, there is still a lack of specialized works on CIC internationally. The publication of this book fills the gap in this field.

This book elaborates on the content and clinical significance of CIC from three aspects: the basic knowledge and procedure methods of CIC, the clinical application of CIC, and the evaluation and follow-up of CIC effects. The book includes the latest new concepts of CIC, such as the application of bladder safe capacity and safe pressure, and the clinical application of partial (morning and evening) CIC, and specifically elaborates on the content of children's CIC. This book is an important reference for healthcare worker, graduate students, undergraduates, especially urologists, pediatric surgeons (pediatric urology), rehabilitation and neurology medical staff, and those engaged in urinary bladder control and ostomy care. Finally, I would like to express my special thanks to my team, my colleagues, and graduate students who have studied and worked together (name list is shown in the end of Foreword). I have consulted a large number of domestic and foreign references, combined with many years of voiding dysfunction diagnosis and treatment and foreign study experience, referred to the ICS and ICCS guidelines, and systematically summarized the knowledge involved in CIC. Zhang Yan and Lv Lei, as the secretaries of this book, have done a lot of coordination work, and I would like to express my thanks here. On the occasion of the publication of this book, I sincerely hope that readers will not hesitate to teach, put forward valuable opinions and suggestions, in order to further improve the future revision, and better serve healthcare worker and patients.

Acknowledgment for their contribution to this book in collecting document and review (in alphabetical order): Chuanchuan Ren, Guanglun Zhou, Jing Yang, Junhua Luo, Lei Lv, Lianghua Jia, Pengchao Xu, Qi Li, Qingwei Wang, Ruili Zhang, Shoulin Li, Wei Zhou, Xinjian Liu, Xuerui Sun, Yan Wang, Yan Zhang, Yulin He

Zhengzhou, China Jian-Guo Wen

Contents

About the Editor

Jian-Guo Wen, M.D., Ph.D., Professor, Chief Physician and Doctoral Supervisor, of Urology/Pediatric Urology, First Affiliated Hospital of Zhengzhou University, and guest professor of First Affiliated Hospital of Xinxiang Medical University, China. He is a special allowances expert of the State Council, outstanding young and middle-aged experts from the Ministry of Health and National level candidates for the "New Century Billion Talents Project," and Honorary Professor of Clinical Medicine, Aarhus University, Denmark.

He received his first doctorate, under the guidance of Professor of Erchang Tong, from Tongji Medical University, China in 1991, and second doctorate, under the guidance of Professor JC Djurhuus, from Aarhus University, Denmark in 2000; he went to Harvard University in the United States for further study in 2004, under the guidance of Professor S.Bauer, former chairman of the International Children's Continence Society (ICCS); in 2009, as the first fully funded (fellowship) urinary bladder control specialist of the International Continence Society (ICS), he went to the Department of Urology at McGill University in Canada for further training, under the guidance of former ICS chairman, Professor J.Corcos. Later, he served as the Vice President of the Pediatric Surgery Physician Branch of the Chinese Medical Doctor Association and the Leader of the Pediatric Urodynamics and Pelvic Floor Group of the Pediatric Surgery Branch of the Chinese Medical Association. He has served as a Committee Member of the Urology Branch of the Chinese Medical Doctor Association. In 2012 and 2013, he was elected as a Urodynamic Committee member, Children and Young Adult's Committee member of the ICS, respectively, and in 2017, he was elected as the first Director of School of Paediatric Voiding Dysfunction and Transitional Urology of ICS; in 2022, he became a Board Member of ICCS.

He has been engaged in urological clinical and scientific research for 40 years and has a deep understanding of the diagnosis and treatment of various voiding dysfunction diseases, especially the diagnosis and treatment of neurogenic bladder (NB). Since 1991, he has published articles on children's NB and pediatric urodynamic study.

He is one of the earliest expert advocates in the treatment of pediatric NB with Clean Intermittent Catheterization (CIC) in China. In 2013, he translated the book *Neurogenic Bladder* edited by J.Corcos, which provides a detailed explanation of how to perform CIC. He is currently leading the National Natural Science Foundation's key projects related to NB, leading his urinary bladder control team to publish more than 700 scientific research papers either in Chinese or in English, and co-editing the world's first pediatric and adolescent urodynamic book (Springer International Publishing AG, 2018) with top international urinary bladder control experts. He has won nine provincial and ministerial level scientific and technological progress awards, including the second prize of the Chinese Medical Science and Technology Award for "Pediatric Bladder Dysfunction and Its Urodynamics Research" (2011). He has obtained 12 invention and utility model patents. In 2013, he won the highest award in the field of urinary bladder control in China, the "Dayu Award." In 2018, he was rated as the first batch of famous doctors in the Central Plains by the Henan Provincial Government. He has actively promoted coprocedure and exchange in the field of medical health between Henan and Denmark and achieved remarkable results, winning the Henan Province International Coprocedure Science and Technology Achievement Award and the highest award for international exchange "Yellow River Friendship Award."

1 The Popularization of Clean Intermittent Catheterization Is a Historical Trend

Jian-Guo Wen

Clean intermittent catheterization (CIC) refers to the method of regularly emptying urine by inserting a catheter into the bladder through the urethra or other bladder outlets (bladder fistula or diversion) under clean conditions [1]. Generally, a disposable sterile catheter is used for catheterization, and the catheter is discarded after voiding. In the past, due to limited medical conditions, catheters were often reused, disinfected after use, and kept for next use, but now they are generally disposable. If reused, the catheter needs to be sterilized by boiling and dried after catheterization and disinfected with iodophor before reuse. The procedure can be completed by the patient himself (clean intermittent self-catheterization) or by family members and caregivers. CIC can protect kidney function and create conditions for patients to participate in social activities for patients with emptying disorders [2, 3].

CIC is also a special catheterization technique, the procedure of which does not require disinfection, just cleanliness. But after all, CIC requires the insertion of a catheter through the urethra for catheterization several times a day, and catheterization is a procedure method that requires certain skills and can easily cause pain and urinary tract infections. In the past, when sanitary conditions were poor, catheter materials were rough, manufacturing technology was backward, and science was not developed. CIC clinical applications are limited. With the development of science and technology and the improvement of sanitary conditions, the popularity rate of CIC is increasing year by year [3].

1.1 The History of Catheterization and CIC

The history of catheterization can be traced back to 3000 BC when Egyptians used flexible gold as a material to make tools for guiding urine. Around 1000 BC, Indian books also described that applying ghee on the surface of a tubular object could lead out urine, which was used to treat urethral stricture and for drug infusion, etc. Erasistos from the Greek island of Kos once used an S-shaped catheter; during the excavation of the ancient city of Pompeii in Italy, a Roman-era metal catheter was also discovered. In addition, reed stalks, rice straw stalks, and tubular objects rolled from palm leaves have all played a role in catheterization [4–6].

The earliest record of catheterization in China is in the Jin Dynasty, Li Shizhen's *Compendium of Materia Medica* Volume 18. Grass Seven "Wang Gua" quoted Jin Ge Hong's "Elbow Back Prescription" saying: "If voiding is not smooth, pound the root of the earth melon into juice, dis-

J.-G. Wen (✉)
Pediatric Urodynamic Center/Department of Urology, First Affiliated Hospital of Zhengzhou University, Zhengzhou, China

J.-G. Wen (ed.), *Progress in Clean Intermittent Catheterization*, Experts' Perspectives on Medical Advances, https://doi.org/10.1007/978-981-97-5021-4_1

solve it in a little water, and blow it into the urethra with a tube." "If defecation is not smooth, blow it into the anus from above; if both voiding and defecation are not smooth, blow it from front and back to make it smooth." This can be said to be the earliest documented catheterization in China. The method recorded in the *Compendium of Materia Medica* is to blow the juice pounded from the root of the earth melon into the urethra with a "tube," using the expansion of the liquid to form a liquid channel and lead out the urine, thus achieving the purpose of catheterization [7]. Although the document does not specify what the catheter is and the process of catheterization, as well as how successful it is, it is enough to prove that catheterization was indeed used clinically at that time. By the Tang Dynasty, a new type of catheterization appeared, and Sun Simiao detailed the method of using onion tube for catheterization. He was also the first person to detail the significance of catheterization. Onion tube catheterization reflects the civilized wisdom of ancient Chinese people. According to Sun Simiao's "Emergency Thousand Gold Recipes," it is recorded: "Whenever urine is not in the bladder, because the bladder is twisted and perverse, the body fluids are not flowing, remove the sharp head with onion leaves, insert into the penis. Three inches deep into the hole, slightly blow it with the mouth, the bladder swells, the body fluids flow greatly and it is cured." This passage detailed the indications for catheterization, catheterization tools, and the depth and specific procedure methods of inserting the catheter into the urethra. In the later Yuan and Ming dynasties, catheterization has greatly improved. The catheters currently widely used in clinical practice originated from some inventions in the Western Middle Ages and later.

Persian philosopher and physician Avicenna designed a bendable urinary tube made of hardened animal skin in 1036, but it did not attract widespread attention. In 1836, French urologist Louis Auguste Mercier made a catheter with a hole in the middle by dipping textile fibers in linseed oil and baking them dry, which greatly facilitated the procedure. After, a Philadelphia businessman Charles Goodyear invented the rubber vulcanization process in 1839; in 1860, Auguste Nélaton, the personal physician of Napoleon III, made a side hole at the top of a red vulcanized rubber tube to create the first rubber catheter. The application of the disinfection method by British doctor Joseph Lister in catheterization reduced the risk of infection, making this procedure more scientific. In 1844, the German Strommeyer first proposed the intermittent catheterization (IC) treatment method, suggesting that infected urine could be expelled by regularly flushing the bladder. In 1940, sterile intermittent catheterization techniques began to be used clinically. In 1947, German scientist Ludwig believed that patients who use catheters for a long time should prefer sterile intermittent catheterization [4–6]. In 1947, Guttmann and others proposed sterile intermittent catheterization (SIC) and recommended it for patients with spinal cord injury (SCI), considered a reasonable bladder management method, avoiding the inconvenience of indwelling catheterization [8].

The SCI patients were catheterized by nurses in the hospital strictly following aseptic procedures. After 11 years of clinical practice of sterile intermittent catheterization, Guttmann's work achieved remarkable achievements in 1966. However, the debate between the supporters and opponents of sterile intermittent catheterization is still very intense. In 1971, American urology professor Lapides found that urinary tract infections during catheterization were due to high pressure and overdistension of the bladder, regardless of the strictness of disinfection. Consequently, he proposed the concept of "clean intermittent catheterization" and pointed out that the measure to prevent infection is to minimize urethral injury. The following year, Lapides advocated clean intermittent self-catheterization (CISC) to treat patients with neurogenic bladder (NB) induced by spinal cord injury [9]. The catheterization procedure is mainly completed by the patient himself. For places lacking personnel and equipment for sterile intermittent catheterization, or for patients who need to do intermittent catheterization at home, CISC is a better choice. Since then, the treatment strategy of NB and urethra dysfunction has fundamentally changed.

IC can help patients avoid long-term indwelling catheters and can maintain periodic expansion and contraction of the bladder and urethral sphincter, allowing urine to be regularly emptied, thereby making the bladder and urethra approach normal physiological functions, gradually restoring the control function of the bladder and sphincter. At the same time, compared with indwelling catheterization, IC can reduce the incidence of urinary tract infections (UTI) [1]. During the First World War, IC was less used, and the mortality rate within a few weeks after spinal cord injury was still as high as 95%, mainly due to urinary retention and sepsis caused by urinary tract infections. Only a few incomplete spinal cord injuries and early reflex voiding survivors survived. During the Second World War, due to the widespread use of IC, the urine handling problem of spinal cord injury patients has made significant progress. Frontline doctors catheterize the bladder of spinal cord injury shock period patients, significantly reducing the number of acute deaths due to urinary tract infections.

In 1960, Lapides discovered that the increase in bladder pressure and urinary retention in patients with NB, rather than the bacteria themselves, were the causes of urinary tract infections. In the winter of 1970, he and nurse Betty Lowe treated a female patient with multiple sclerosis for the first time using CIC; the patient achieved urinary bladder control, and no urinary tract infection occurred in a short period, and this simple and convenient catheterization technique did not produce any adverse reactions. In 1972, Lapides and others proposed CIC treatment for neurogenic bladder (NB), quickly becoming a life-saving treatment measure for those NB patients who cannot empty their bladder autonomously. CIC can prevent excessive bladder expansion, prevent abnormal increase in bladder pressure, increase blood circulation in the bladder wall, and enhance the bladder mucosa's resistance to infection [9]. SIC can only be implemented in the hospital; if SIC is to be carried out after discharge, it will inevitably bring great inconvenience to discharged patients and even affect the quality of life of patients. Kessler and others evaluated patients who had used CIC for more than 5 years, suggesting that 80% of patients believe that CIC is relatively easy and does not interfere with daily life. Before CIC was widely used in the treatment of NB, renal failure and uremia were common causes of death in patients. Fortunately, with the gradual implementation of CIC, it has achieved significant therapeutic effects in preventing vesicoureteral reflux (VUR) and hydronephrosis, reducing the rate of bladder enlargement surgery, and reducing postoperative deaths due to renal failure.

With the development of technology, various indications and complications of CIC are gradually being recognized and summarized, so that it can be better applied to patients. The application of CIC can regularly store and discharge urine, restore bladder function, and avoid various complications caused by long-term indwelling catheterization such as urinary tract infections, bladder stones, urethral injuries, urinary retention after catheter removal, urethral external ulcer, etc.

The widespread use of CIC is inseparable from the continuous progress of catheter material and design. New technologies and materials are constantly emerging, and the material and design of catheters are also being updated accordingly. The selection of a CIC catheter must take into account the patient's actual condition, such as the degree of injury, hand function, degree of visual impairment, sensitivity of the urethra, gender, age, economic status, and other related factors. Patients often need to try several different types of catheters before making a final choice. Clinical nurses need to understand the characteristics of various types of catheters in order to guide patients to make correct and reasonable choices.

In the twentieth and twenty-first centuries, new materials such as latex, synthetic rubber, and silicone have emerged, bringing many durable products to people. In the 1930s, Frederic Foley invented a rubber catheter with a tube inside to inflate a small sac to fix the catheter in the bladder. The initial catheter was an open system, where the urine in the catheter dripped into an open container, which greatly relieved the patient's pain, but 100% of patients with this type of catheter would get an infection within 4 days or longer. In the 1950s, a closed catheter system appeared, where urine could flow down the catheter into a sealed bag. Modern types of catheters include uncoated catheters, coated catheters, and closed systems, which have greatly reduced the incidence of CIC complications [4, 10].

The CIC technology widely used in Europe and America has little impact on the patient's life and does not require long-term carrying of a urine bag, thus improving the quality of life of the patient, which is of great significance in helping patients lead a normal life. Especially for children with NB, if the bladder cannot be emptied in time, the increased bladder pressure will cause damage to the upper urinary tract. Even if the child's cognitive ability or behavioral ability does not meet the requirements, if the parents learn and help the child operate, CIC can be performed. After more than 40 years of development, CIC has been recognized by the International Continence Society (ICS) as the preferred treatment method for emptying the bladder, which can effectively empty the bladder and is gradually being applied in clinical practice [11]. The application of CIC in China is not as widespread as abroad, and there are few literature reports on CIC, especially in children. The monograph on CIC is still lacking and needs to continue to strive to keep pace with the international community.

1.2 Reasons Why Clean Intermittent Catheterization Is a Historical Trend

The author believes that the popularization of CIC is a historical trend. The reasons are as follows: (1) Patients who need CIC are mostly those with NB and low detrusor function, and many patients have lost their ability to urinate. The treatment of these diseases is still a world difficult problem, and there is no effective cure. (2) The current treatment methods are mostly symptomatic treatment, and CIC is the simplest and most effective treatment method. (3) The continuous improvement and progress of catheter materials and manufacturing processes have significantly reduced the pain and complications caused by CIC. (4) With the development of modern networks and technological progress, the popularization and training of knowledge on CIC have significantly improved. (5) The advancement of bladder function evaluation techniques such as urodynamic study, as well as the introduction of new concepts and theories such as bladder safe capacity, safe pressure, and catheterization diary, has laid the foundation for more precise and safe catheterization. (6) The popularization of hand hygiene knowledge and the emergence of effective antibiotics have effectively prevented and treated CIC-related urinary tract infections. (7) With the deepening understanding of newborn NB, starting CIC from the newborn period has been written into the guidelines of the European Association of Urology (EAU) [12], part (early and late) catheterization effectively improved enuresis and nocturia and improved bladder control ability, significantly expanding the application range of CIC.

References

1. Prieto JA, Murphy CL, Stewart F, Fader M. Intermittent catheter techniques, strategies and designs for managing long-term bladder conditions [J]. Cochrane Database Syst Rev. 2021;10(10):CD006008.
2. Wang J, Feng M, Liao T, et al. Effects of clean intermittent catheterization and transurethral indwelling catheterization on the management of urinary retention after gynecological surgery: a systematic review and meta-analysis [J]. Transl Androl Urol. 2023;12(5):744–60.
3. Elliott CS. Sustainability in urology: single-use versus reusable catheters for intermittent catheterization [J]. Eur Urol Focus. 2023;9(6):888–90. https://doi.org/10.1016/j.euf.2023.09.012.
4. Bloom DA, Mcguire EJ, Lapides J. A brief history of urethral catheterization [J]. J Urol. 1994;151(2):317–25. https://doi.org/10.1016/s0022-5347(17)34937-6.
5. Feneley RC, Hopley IB, Wells PN. Urinary catheters: history, current status, adverse events and research agenda [J]. J Med Eng Technol. 2015;39(8):459–70. https://doi.org/10.3109/03091902.2015.1085600.
6. Wang B, Zhao X. The invention and development of catheterization [J]. Chin Nurs Res. 2008;(31):2913. [王斌全，赵晓云. 导尿术的发明与发展. 护理研究，2008;(31):2913].
7. Du Y. A brief history of the application of catheterization in ancient China [J]. Chin J Med Hist.

1995;25(1):35–7. [杜勇. 中国古代导尿术应用史略. 中华医史杂志, 1995;25(1):35–7].
8. Guttmann L, Riches EW, Whitteridge D, et al. Discussion on the treatment and prognosis of traumatic paraplegia [J]. Proc R Soc Med. 1947;40(5):219–32.
9. Lapides J, Diokno AC, Silber SJ, Lowe BS. Clean, intermittent self-catheterization in the treatment of urinary tract disease [J]. J Urol. 1972;107(3):458–61.
10. Patel SR, Caldamone AA. The history of urethral catheterization [J]. Med Health R I. 2004;87(8):240–2.
11. D'Ancona C, Haylen B, Oelke M, et al. The International Continence Society (ICS) report on the terminology for adult male lower urinary tract and pelvic floor symptoms and dysfunction [J]. Neurourol Urodyn. 2019;38(2):433–77. https://doi.org/10.1002/nau.23897.
12. Stein R, Bogaert G, Dogan HS, et al. EAU/ESPU guidelines on the management of neurogenic bladder in children and adolescent part I diagnostics and conservative treatment [J]. Neurourol Urodyn. 2020;39(1):45–57. https://doi.org/10.1002/nau.24211.

2 Knowledge of Urinary System Anatomy Is the Basis of CIC

Jian-Guo Wen

CIC requires understanding of the anatomy and pathophysiology of the urinary system, especially the location and morphology of the urethral orifice, and the characteristics of different ages and genders.

The anatomy related to CIC, especially the anatomical characteristics of the urethra and bladder of different age groups, is essential for successfully completing CIC. Successful catheterization first requires finding the correct urethral orifice and smoothly inserting the catheter into the urethra, while minimizing damage to the urethral mucosa as much as possible. Therefore, it is necessary to understand the anatomical features such as the course and physiological curvature of the urethra. The following introduces the anatomical features of the urethra and bladder related to different genders and age groups, hoping to provide help for health-care worker and patients to perform CIC.

2.1 Urethral Anatomy and Physiology

When we perform intermittent catheterization, the catheter first enters the bladder through the urethra. How to correctly find the external urethral orifice? How to smoothly insert the catheter into the urethra and minimize irritation and damage to the urethra? To solve these problems, we first need to understand the basic anatomy of the urethra, including the characteristics of the urethra in different genders and age groups; catheterization can be performed according to different characteristics during catheterization, enhancing patient compliance with catheterization, thereby helping patients to complete CIC more safely and efficiently.

2.1.1 Anatomy of the Male Urethra [1]

2.1.1.1 Morphology and Structure

The male urethra is a long tubular organ that originates from the bladder neck and ends at the external urethral orifice at the top of the penis. It only has a voiding function at the beginning and also has an ejaculation function after puberty. The fetal male urethra begins to develop at 8 weeks of embryonic gestation.

The fetal kidney begins to produce urine, and fetal voiding can be detected by ultrasound at 20 weeks of gestation. The growth of the male newborn urethra is slow, and it grows rapidly after puberty.

At the age of 1 year, the length of the male urethra is 5–6 cm, and the length is about 12 cm at sexual maturity. The male urethra is divided into three parts: the prostatic part, the membra-

J.-G. Wen (✉)
Pediatric Urodynamic Center/Department of Urology, First Affiliated Hospital of Zhengzhou University, Zhengzhou, China

J.-G. Wen (ed.), *Progress in Clean Intermittent Catheterization*, Experts' Perspectives on Medical Advances, https://doi.org/10.1007/978-981-97-5021-4_2

nous part, and the spongy part. Clinically, the prostatic part and the membranous part are generally referred to as the posterior urethra, and the spongy part is referred to as the anterior urethra.

Prostatic part: The prostatic part of the urethra is the part of the urethra that passes through the prostate, starting from the internal urethral orifice and ending at the tip of the prostate, closest to the front of the prostate. There is a longitudinal bulge on the posterior wall of this part of the urethra, called the urethral crest; the bulging part in the crest is called the seminal colliculus, and there is a small depression in the center of the seminal colliculus, called the prostatic utricle, which is the remnant of the degeneration of the distal side of the accessory mesonephric duct, with no physiological function.

Membranous part: The membranous part is the part of the urethra that passes through the urogenital diaphragm, located between the prostate and the bulbous urethra, extending forward from the back, and is the narrowest part of the three sections. It is surrounded by the urethral sphincter, which is a striated muscle that controls voiding, also known as the external urethral sphincter. Although the membranous urethra is small, it is highly expandable and appears star-shaped on the cross-section of the urethra. However, due to the thin wall of this section of the urethra and the fixation of surrounding tissues such as the puboprostatic ligament and the periurethral fascia, it is prone to injury when the pelvic bone is fractured. The junction with the spongy part of the urethra has the weakest wall, surrounded only by loose connective tissue, and is prone to injury when inserting instruments into the urethra.

Spongy part: The spongy part is the longest section of the urethra and the least developed part in newborns. It starts at the end of the membranous urethra and ends at the external urethral orifice, running through the entire urethral spongiosum. The starting part of this section of the urethra is inside the urethral bulb, which is the widest part of the entire urethra, known as the bulbous urethra. The bulbourethral glands open here, and straddle injuries often damage this area. The middle part of the urethral spongiosum is relatively narrow, with a diameter of about 0.6 cm, and at the end of the glans penis, it expands into a navicular fossa. From the navicular fossa to the external urethral orifice, the urethral lumen gradually narrows again, forming one of the narrow parts of the urethra. The diameter of the external urethral orifice in children is about 0.5 cm.

The male urethra varies in width, with three narrowings, three expansions, and two bends. The three narrowings are located at the internal urethral orifice, the membranous urethra, and the external urethral orifice, with the membranous part being the narrowest. Urethral stones often get stuck in these narrow areas. The three expansions are located in the prostatic part of the urethra, the bulbous part of the urethra, and the navicular fossa of the urethra, with the navicular fossa being the largest, the bulbous part second, and the prostatic part the smallest. The two bends are the infrapubic bend protruding downward and backward and the prepubic bend protruding upward and forward. The infrapubic bend is fixed and located about 2 cm below the pubic symphysis, including the prostatic part of the urethra, the membranous part, and the starting segment of the spongy part, forming a bend that protrudes backward. The prepubic bend is located in front and below the front of symphysis, between the root and body of the penis. When the penis is erect or lifted upward, this bend can straighten and disappear. Figure 2.1 is a sagittal view of the male pelvis published by Vishy Mahadevan in 2019 in "Anatomy of the lower urinary tract," showing the course of the male urethra and its relationship with the bladder [2].

The tissue structure of the prostate, membranous, and spongy parts of the male child's urethra is different, and the urethra wall can be divided into the mucosal layer, submucosal layer, and muscle layer. The urethral epithelial cells are developed from the epithelial cells of the inner embryonic layer. The prostate part of the urethra is covered by transitional epithelium, which can extend into the prostate gland duct. The epithelium of the membranous part of the urethra is columnar, either stratified or pseudostratified, and the proximal part of the spongy urethra is covered by stratified or pseudostratified colum-

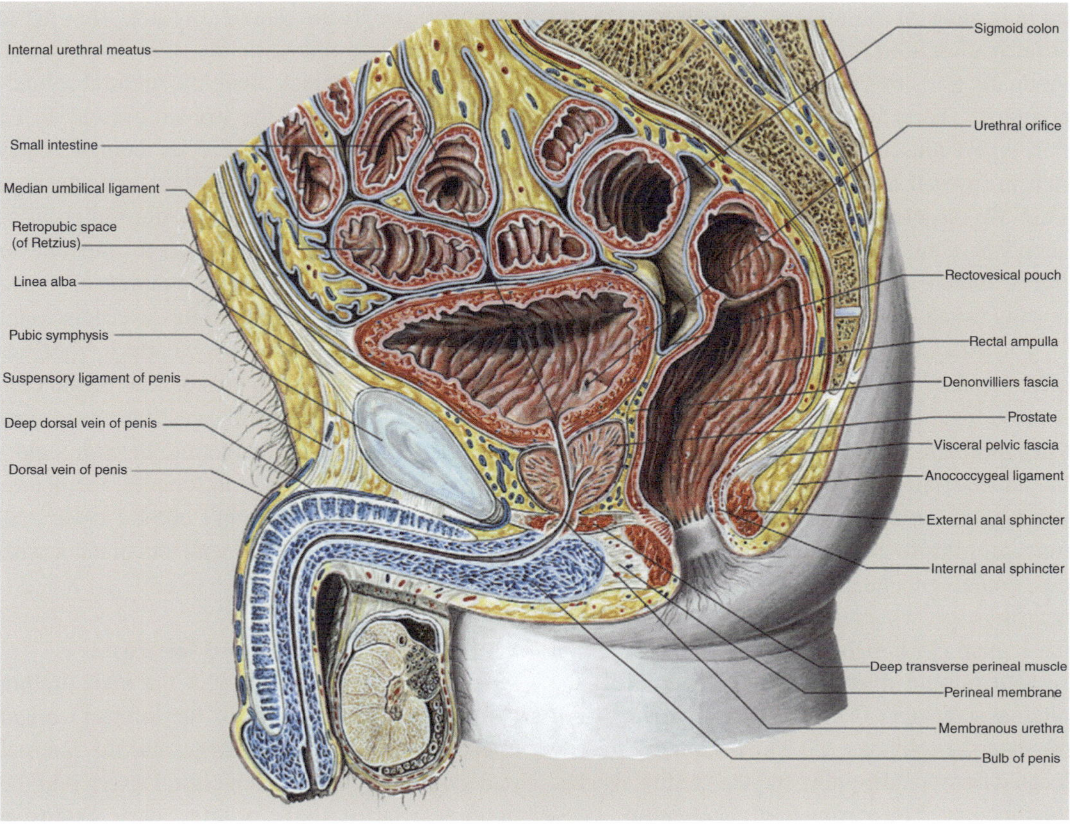

Fig. 2.1 Sagittal view of the male pelvis ("Anatomy of the lower urinary tract" come from Vishy Mahadevan [2])

nar epithelium. The distal part is covered by stratified squamous epithelium. The mucosal propria is formed by loose connective tissue, containing a rich network of elastic fibers and blood vessels. The boundary between the submucosal layer of the urethra and the propria is not clear, and it is also loose connective tissue. The development of the newborn's urethral mucosa is poor, the mucosal epithelium is easy to fall off and get injured, and the development of the mucosal glands, elastic fibers, and connective tissue is also poor.

The muscle layer of the prostate part of the urethra is surrounded by an inner longitudinal and an outer circular smooth muscle layer. The small glands around the urethra can extend into the longitudinal smooth muscle fibers and terminate at the external sphincter.

The membranous part of the urethra not only contains inner longitudinal and outer circular smooth muscle layers but is also surrounded by an external sphincter. The external sphincter is often mistakenly described as a flat muscle sandwiched between two layers of fascia like a sandwich. The external sphincter is actually ring-shaped, with a wide base, narrowing at the upper part and merging with the tip of the prostate through the urogenital hiatus above the levator ani. During embryonic development, these muscles form a vertical tube extending from the membranous urethra to the neck of the bladder. With the development of the prostate, the muscles on the posterior and lateral sides gradually atrophy, while the transverse muscle fibers in front of the prostate remain intact until adulthood. The ring-shaped muscle fibers at the tip of the prostate surround the urethra, and the muscle fibers at the back of the urethra are thinner and merge into a fibrous sheath. At the distal end, these muscle fibers do not merge at the back of the urethra but form an Ω shape, only distributed on both sides of the urethra; smooth muscle and striated muscle in the middle 1/3 of the urethra gradually transition to form the urethral sphincter complex. The external sphincter is composed of thin type I muscle fibers (slow response fibers), rich in myosin adenosine triphosphatase, which keep the muscles in a contracted state. There is abundant connective tissue around the muscle fibers, which is connected to the adjacent supporting tissue [3, 4].

The external sphincter corresponds to the maximum urethral closure pressure, and its voiding control function disappears after prostatectomy. The mechanisms of urethral closure pressure include the following: (1) The contraction of pseudostratified columnar epithelium forms radial mucosal folds to close the lumen. (2) The submucosa contains abundant blood vessels and soft connective tissue, which is conducive to the closure of the lumen. (3) Longitudinal and circular urethral smooth muscle fibers (the inner part forms the internal sphincter). (4) The contraction function of the external sphincter. (5) The levator ani muscle located between the pubis and the urethra also has the function of increasing urethral pressure.

The muscle layer of the spongy urethra only has one layer of circular smooth muscle, but the urethral glands in this part are significantly increased compared to the prostate and membranous parts. The urethral gland is a mucous gland, formed by the cup-shaped cells scattered on the surface of the urethral mucosal epithelium sinking into the pits, growing, and extending to the deep surface of the mucosa. The glandular epithelium is columnar, and the cytoplasm is clear and contains mucous granules.

The pelvic plexus sends branches to the prostate and important penile cavernous nerves near the tail part. After passing through the tip of the seminal vesicle, these nerves are located in the lateral leaf of the pelvic fascia but run laterally on the surface of the rectum at the postero-lateral edge of the prostate, lateral to the prostatic venous plexus. Because these nerves are composed of numerous nerve fibers, they are not easily distinguishable to the naked eye, but blood vessels are often surgical markers for recognizing nerve pathways (Walsh's vascular nerve bundle). After reaching the membranous urethra, the nerve divides into two branches, the superficial branch runs at 3 and 9 o'clock along the urethral sphincter and infiltrates into the striated muscle of the urethral sphincter, and the deep branch issues small branches to the bulbourethral gland through this muscle. When reaching the starting point of the penis, these nerves will merge into one to three separate nerve bundles, running at 1 and 11 o'clock, on the surface of the cavernous vein, the dorsal side of the cavernous artery. Together with the artery, they pass through the penile cavernous body to control the erection tissue, and small nerve fibers also merge into the penile dorsal nerve at the distal end. In females, the nerves controlling the vestibule and clitoral cavernous body run along the vaginal wall and bladder with the lateral venous plexus.

2.1.1.2 Blood Vessels and Nerves

Arteries: The arterial supply of the male urethra comes from the branches of the inferior vesical artery, the inferior rectal artery, and the internal pudendal artery (the bulbourethral artery and the urethral artery); these arteries have extensive communicating branches. The arteries of the penis mainly include two dorsal penile arteries and two deep penile arteries, all of which are terminal branches of the penile artery. In the process of the dorsal penile artery running to the glans, it gives off branches to the penile cavernous body and the urethral cavernous body. The rich blood supply of the urethral cavernous body allows urologists to free the urethra in the repair surgery of urethral stricture.

Veins: The veins of the urethra mainly drain into the vesical venous plexus and the pudendal venous plexus and finally into the internal iliac vein.

Nerves: The urethra is mainly controlled by the pudendal nerve, which includes branches of the perineal nerve, sympathetic nerve, and parasympathetic nerve. The prostate is controlled by sympathetic and parasympathetic nerves originating from the pelvic plexus. The nerves and arteries enter the prostate and stroma at right angles. The parasympathetic nerves terminate in the acini and control their secretion, while the sympathetic nerve fibers control the contraction of the smooth muscles in the prostate capsule and stroma. The α1 blockers can relax the tension of the prostate stroma and the peri-prostatic sphincter, improving the flow rate in patients with prostate hyperplasia. The efferent nerves of the prostate reach the pelvic and thoracolumbar spinal nerve centers through the pelvic nerves. The nerves of the membranous urethral sphincter are controlled by the sacral nerves two to four segments and branches of the pudendal nerve. The autonomic nerves that control the inner smooth muscle of the membranous urethra may originate from the cavernous nerves, but their role in controlling voiding is not significant. The efferent nerves of the external sphincter are still unclear, but it can be confirmed that they play a significant role. Gross anatomy and retrograde axonal tracing techniques have confirmed that the external sphincter of the membranous urethra is controlled by the pudendal nerve, but what has always puzzled urologists is why cutting the pudendal nerve cannot stop the contraction of the external sphincter [5, 6].

2.1.2 Anatomy of the Female Urethra [1]

2.1.2.1 Morphology and Structure

The female urethra only has a voiding function, starting from the internal urethral orifice, passing through the urogenital diaphragm in front of the vagina, and ending at the external urethral orifice. The external urethral orifice is exposed and close to the anus, easily contaminated by feces, and retrograde infections are more common than in males. When passing through the urogenital diaphragm, it is surrounded by the urethrovaginal sphincter. The characteristic of female urethra is one of the reasons why urinary tract infections are more common in females than in males. Above the urogenital diaphragm, there is a pudendal venous plexus between the front of the urethra and the pubic symphysis, and the back of the urethra is closely connected to the front wall of the vagina through loose connective tissue. The tissue between the urethra and the vagina is called the urethrovaginal septum. The front and sides of the part below the urogenital diaphragm are adjacent to the junction of the two clitoral legs. The female internal urethral orifice is similar to the male, and the external orifice is a sagittal slit; the surrounding area is raised and papillary, located in front of the vaginal orifice behind the clitoris. The suspensory ligament of the clitoris (anterior urethral ligament) and the pubourethral ligament (posterior urethral ligament) form a sling to suspend the urethra on the pubis. Figure 2.2 is a sagittal view of the female pelvis published by Vishy Mahadevan in 2019 in "Anatomy of the lower urinary tract," showing the relationship between the female urethra and the vagina [2].

2.1.2.2 Tissue Structure

The female urethra is composed of mucosa and muscle layers, with a thick inherent layer and rich mucosa, often forming urethral mucosal folds. The surface of the urethra is covered with transitional epithelium and non-keratinized squamous epithelium. Many small mucosal glands open into the urethra, easily forming urethral diverticula. At the distal end of the urethra, these glands gather on both sides of the urethra into groups (group glands), which are emptied through gland ducts that open together at the urethral orifice. The muscle layer consists of inner longitudinal and outer circular layers. A thin, vascular-rich mucosal muscle layer supports the urethra and glands. These structures all depend on estrogen, and atrophy occurs after menopause, leading to stress urinary incontinence [7, 8]. A relatively weak layer of longitudinal smooth muscle runs from the neck of the bladder to the external urethral orifice, entering the fat and fibrous tissue around the urethra. Unlike the proximal urethra in males, the female proximal urethra does not have a circular sphincter, and its posterior wall muscle fibers are relatively lacking. A thinner layer of circular smooth muscle wraps around the longitudinal muscle layer, extending the full length of the urethra. During voiding, the longitudinal muscles and detrusor contract simultaneously, making the urethra shorter and wider. The striated muscle fibers of the proximal 1/3 of the female fetus's urethra are relatively less distributed, with myelinated and

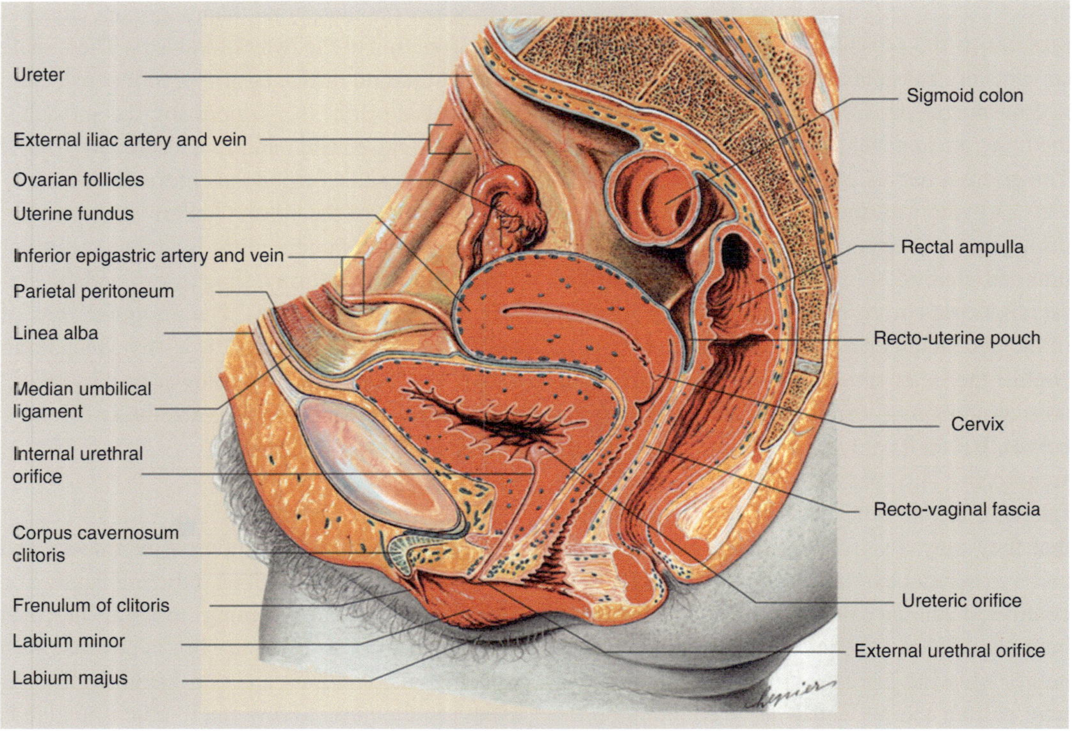

Fig. 2.2 Sagittal view of the female pelvis ("Anatomy of the lower urinary tract" come from Vishy Mahadevan [2])

unmyelinated nerve fibers running on the posterior surface of the proximal 1/3 of the urethra, controlling the smooth muscle fibers [4].

The external sphincter is located at the distal 2/3 of the urethra. It is composed of type I muscle fibers (slow reactive fibers), surrounded by abundant collagen tissue. The external sphincter can completely encircle the urethra, playing an important role in the maximum closure pressure of the urethra. The muscle fibers do not converge at the back of the urethra after passing the urethra but continue from both sides of the urethra to the anterior and lateral walls of the vagina. These muscle fibers completely encircle the urethra and vagina to form the urethrovaginal sphincter. These muscles contract together with the bulbospongiosus muscle, tightening the urogenital hiatus [3].

2.1.2.3 Blood Vessels and Nerves

The arteries of the female urethra mainly come from the branches of the inferior vesical artery, uterine artery, and pudendal artery (vestibular artery of the vagina and urethral artery); these arteries have extensive anastomoses with each other. The urethral veins drain into the vesical venous plexus and pudendal venous plexus, finally entering the internal iliac vein. The nerves of the female urethra are controlled by the pudendal nerve, sympathetic nerve, and parasympathetic nerve. Its external urethral sphincter receives dual somatic nerve innervation, like males, receiving innervation from the pudendal and pelvic somatic nerves. A small amount of sympathetic nerves can also be found in the female urethra. Cholinergic nerve fibers of the parasympathetic system are found in the smooth muscles. Somatic and autonomic nerve plexuses run along the vaginal sidewall adjacent to the urethra. During stress urinary incontinence surgery through the vagina, these nerves should be avoided when incising the anterior vaginal wall to prevent the occurrence of type III urinary incontinence [5, 7, 9].

2.1.3 Urethral Anatomy Characteristics in Different Age Groups

2.1.3.1 Anatomical Characteristics of the Children

The anatomical characteristics of the pediatric urinary system are that the bladder is located higher, the newborn bladder is often pear-shaped and located above the pubic symphysis, and the infant bladder is close to the anterior abdominal wall and gradually descends into the pelvic cavity with age [10]. The urethra of male newborns and infants is short and delicate. Conditions such as phimosis and excessive foreskin, which are not conducive to displaying the urethral orifice, are common, and it is not easy to expose the urethral orifice. When performing CIC procedures, care should be taken to gently peel back the foreskin to expose the urethral orifice, gently insert a thinner catheter, and avoid damaging the urethra to the greatest extent possible. Special attention should be paid to foreskin cleanliness. The urethra of a 1-year-old boy is 5–6 cm long and about 12 cm at puberty. Male infants often have phimosis or excessive foreskin at birth. The foreskin is often not completely free from the glans penis, but is physiologically adhered. As the penis develops with age, the adhesion gradually separates and absorbs, and the foreskin retracts on its own. Generally, by the age of 10, 2–3% of males still have phimosis. Male infants with phimosis are prone to accumulation of smegma, which can easily lead to ascending bacterial infections. If long-term CIC is required, a circumcision procedure is needed.

The characteristics of the urethra in female newborns and infants are that the urethra is short and delicate, the labia minora are prone to adhesion, and the urethral orifice is often difficult to identify. The urethra of a female newborn is only 1 cm and can later increase to 3–5 cm. When performing CIC procedures, be gentle, soothe the child's emotions, maintain cleanliness, and avoid urethral injury and infection.

2.1.3.2 Anatomical Characteristics of the Urethra in Young Adults

The urethra of a young adult male is 17–20 cm long, with two bends, the prepubic bend and the infrapubic bend, and three narrow parts, the external orifice, the membranous part, and the internal orifice. These anatomical characteristics should be taken into account when inserting the catheter. The penis should be lifted to form a 60° angle with the abdominal wall to eliminate the prepubic bend, allowing the catheter to be inserted smoothly. The depth should be about 20 cm, and once urine starts to flow, insert another 2 cm. In addition, considering the anatomical characteristics of the male urethra, a curved catheter can be chosen, which is easier to insert.

The characteristics of the urethra in young adult females are as follows:

1. The female urethral orifice is located below the clitoris and above the vaginal orifice and is thick and short. The length of the urethra in adult females is usually 3–5 cm. When performing CIC, gently insert the catheter 4–6 cm, and once urine starts to flow, insert another 1 cm.
2. Some female patients, due to childbirth or the rupture of the hymen, may have more skin folds around the urethral orifice, making it difficult to locate the external urethral orifice during catheterization.
3. Women are prone to urethral syndrome [11]. Urethral syndrome refers to a group of nonspecific syndromes characterized by symptoms such as frequent voiding, urgency, and pain during voiding, but no significant organic changes are found in the bladder and urethra upon examination. It is more common in married middle-aged women. It is often caused by anatomical abnormalities of the external urethral orifice (such as labial fusion, urethral hymen fusion, hymen umbrella, etc.), distal urethral obstruction, urinary system infection, and local chemical and mechanical stimulation. There may be mucosal edema and urethral secretions at the external urethral ori-

fice, and sometimes urethral polyps, urethral hymen fusion, and hymen umbrella can be seen. There is tenderness in the urethra and bladder neck accompanied by urethral induration. These symptoms will affect the exposure of the urethra during catheterization and the insertion of the catheter.

4. The female urethral orifice is not as visible as the male's, and it is adjacent to the vaginal orifice, making it easy to mistakenly insert the catheter into the vagina, especially for women when self-catheterizing, and beginners often need to use a mirror to successfully locate the urethral orifice [12].

2.1.3.3 Anatomical Characteristics of the Urethra in the Elderly

Middle-aged and elderly male patients often have varying degrees of prostatic hyperplasia, which can cause significant resistance when inserting a catheter. Prostatic hyperplasia is actually the gradual enlargement of the glandular tissue, connective tissue, and smooth muscle tissue around the posterior urethra from the bladder neck to the perineum under the influence of α-dihydrotestosterone. The enlarging nodules continuously expand, compressing the outer glandular tissue into a so-called "pseudocapsule" or "surgical capsule" that is 2–5 mm thick. The enlarged prostate protrudes into the posterior urethra and bladder neck, sometimes protruding into the bladder, changing the normal anatomical shape of the posterior urethra, thereby causing the urethra to be compressed, elongated, and narrowed and the bladder neck to become smaller, leading to urinary obstruction. This can cause a series of pathological changes in the parts above the posterior urethra. If not treated in time, it can affect kidney function, leading to chronic renal failure, uremia, and other serious consequences [13].

Proper adjustment of the catheter insertion method and penile position can help patients with prostatic hyperplasia insert the catheter. Especially for patients after transurethral resection of the prostate, their urethra often has a lot of scar tissue, making the urethral wall rough and irregular, so the key points of catheter insertion should be paid more attention to.

Patients with prostatic hyperplasia have more difficulty in catheterization than general male patients, which can easily cause damage to the urethral mucosa and cause bleeding. Under the guidance of a professional doctor, paying attention to the technique of inserting the catheter can alleviate the patient's pain and increase the success rate of one-time catheterization.

2.2 Bladder Anatomy and Physiology

The bladder is an organ that stores urine, which is excreted from the body through the urethra. Understanding the anatomy and physiological characteristics of the bladder can help patients better choose the timing of catheterization, the appropriate interval between catheterizations, and the amount of urine to be drained each time.

2.2.1 The Shape and Adjacency of the Bladder

The bladder is a conical muscular organ that stores urine. Its size, shape, and position vary with age and its filling state. The infant bladder is spindle-shaped and located higher than in adults. When filled with urine, it can rise into the abdominal cavity and can be palpated above the pubic symphysis. Its neck is close to the upper edge of the pubic symphysis. As age increases, due to the expansion of the pubic bone, the enlargement of the pelvic cavity, the evolution of the sacral angle, and the tilt and depth of the pelvis, the bladder gradually descends into the pelvis, reaching the adult position around puberty [2, 5].

The newborn bladder is spindle-shaped or pear-shaped when not filled and round when filled, similar to adults. The empty bladder can be divided into four parts, body, bottom, top, and neck, but there is no clear boundary between each part. The bladder has an upper, posterior, and two lower lateral surfaces: the upper surface is triangular, with the two lateral edges being the line from the top to the lateral angle and the posterior edge being the line between the two lateral angles; the posterior of the bladder, also known as the bladder base, is triangular and faces the posterior inferior direction; the lower lateral surface faces the anterior lateral inferior direction and is connected to the pelvic diaphragm; the large part between the top and bottom of the bladder is called the bladder body; the lowest part of the bladder, i.e., the meeting point of the posterior and left and right lower lateral edges, is called the bladder neck. The male bladder neck is connected to the prostate, while the female is connected to the urethra and pelvic diaphragm. The meeting point of the upper, lower lateral, and bottom surfaces of the bladder is the lateral angle, slightly below which is where the ureter enters the bladder. Inside the bladder, there are two openings connected to the ureters, called the ureteral openings. The bladder wall bulges between the lines connecting the two ureteral openings, called the ureteral ridge. The bladder outlet is composed of the bladder base, urethra, and external urethral sphincter. The lower part of the lower lateral side of the bladder is adjacent to the levator ani muscle, and its lower lateral side is connected to the levator ani, obturator internus, and the loose connective tissue between their fascia, called the paravesical tissue.

The thickness of the bladder muscle layer changes with the degree of bladder distension. It is thickest in the bladder trigone area, where the inner muscle layer is a submucosal muscle (trigone muscle) different from the intrinsic muscle of the bladder wall, formed by the extension of the longitudinal muscle layer of the left and right ureters to the urethra and each other, reaching the prostatic vesicles through the posterior wall of the urethra. When the bladder contracts, many folds are formed on the inner surface, which completely disappear when it expands, while the bladder trigone has no folds whether it is expanded or contracted.

The female bladder differs from the male bladder in the following ways: the base of the female bladder does not have a peritoneum, and it is adjacent to the anterior wall of the vagina and the cervix through the loose connective tissue rich in veins, forming the bladder-vaginal septum. The upper and lower outer lateral surfaces of the bladder are covered with peritoneum, which moves upward with the filling of urine. The posterior edge of the bladder corresponds to the plane of the internal orifice of the uterus, its surface is covered with peritoneum, and it moves backward and upward, located in front of the body of the uterus above it. The peritoneum folds back between the bladder and the uterus to form the bladder-uterine depression. Most of the lower outer lateral surface of the bladder is not covered with peritoneum, and the round ligament of the uterus passes nearby. The sides of the bladder anterior space are the pubic bladder ligaments, the neck of the bladder is directly connected to the urogenital diaphragm, and it is connected to the urethra downward [4].

2.2.2 Tissue Structure of the Bladder

The bladder wall is divided into three layers: the bladder mucosa, the bladder muscle layer, and the bladder serosa.

2.2.2.1 Bladder Mucosa

The bladder mucosa is rich, wrinkled when empty, and flattened when filled; wrinkles disappear.

The mucosal epithelium is transitional epithelium, and the number of layers is related to function and location. When the bladder contracts, the epithelium thickens to six to eight layers, the surface cells are large cuboidal, and there are one to two cell nucleus; when the bladder is filled, the epithelium becomes thinner, the cell layer is reduced to two to three layers, and the surface cells become flat. The basement membrane is not obvious, the proper membrane is dense connective tissue, there are a small number of lymph nodes in the mucosa, and the deep tissue of the mucosa is loose, like the submucosa. Electron microscopy observes that the free surface of the mucosal epithelial surface layer cells has many densely arranged tiny wrinkles and grooves, the cytoplasm is dispersed in the shallow layer, and there are fusiform or tubular vesicles. The outer side of the surface membrane is thickened, and frozen specimens find that protein particles in this layer of membrane are gathered and densely arranged, while the inner side particles are dispersed, and bundles of microfilaments are distributed in the cytoplasm directly below the inner side, forming a shell layer. The tops of adjacent cells are tightly connected; with more connections and dense networks, this structure is the barrier of the bladder mucosa to prevent the penetration of large molecules. The base of the cell has densely arranged membrane folds to adapt to the contraction and expansion of the bladder [14].

2.2.2.2 Bladder Muscle Layer

The bladder muscle layer is thick, and the connective tissue between the muscle bundles is rich. The muscle fibers criss-cross, but it can be roughly divided into three layers: the outer longitudinal, middle circular, and inner longitudinal. At the internal orifice of the urethra, the middle layer muscle fibers thicken to form the internal urethral sphincter. The bladder muscle layer contains a rich supply of parasympathetic nerve fibers. The length of the detrusor fibers varies greatly, generating tension by using the extracellular matrix as a fulcrum, thereby causing bladder contraction.

2.2.2.3 Bladder Serosa

The bladder serosa is mainly fibrous, with loosely arranged fibers, containing blood vessels, nerves, and lymphatic vessels. The upper back of the bladder is a serous membrane.

2.2.3 Blood Vessels and Nerve Supply of the Bladder

The bladder arteries are divided into superior, middle, and inferior bladder arteries. The superior and inferior bladder arteries originate from the anterior trunk of the internal iliac artery, and the middle artery originates from the internal iliac artery. There are also bladder branches from the obturator artery and the inferior gluteal artery. In females, there are branches from the uterine artery and the vaginal artery. The bladder veins do not accompany their arteries and form a rich venous plexus in the bladder wall or on its surface. These veins form a bladder venous plexus or a bladder-prostate venous plexus on the lower outer side of the bladder and on both sides of the prostate, which drains into the internal iliac vein. The bladder venous plexus communicates posteriorly with the rectal venous plexus, and in females, it communicates with the uterovaginal venous plexus; anteriorly, it communicates with the genital veins; therefore, during bladder resection, if the bladder venous plexus is not securely ligated, it can cause severe bleeding.

The bladder is innervated by the autonomic nerves, with nerve fibers composed of sympathetic nerves from the inferior mesenteric ganglion and parasympathetic nerve fibers from the sacral cord two to four forming the bladder plexus [6]. This nerve plexus is divided into the paravesical plexus located on both sides of the bladder and the intrinsic bladder nerve plexus within the bladder wall. The bladder is mainly innervated by the parasympathetic nerves, which cause contraction of the bladder muscle layer, while the sympathetic nerve fibers in the muscle layer are scarce, causing relaxation of the muscle layer. The bladder neck and posterior urethra are mainly innervated by the sympathetic nerves, causing contraction of the bladder neck [15]. The genital nerves are directly controlled by consciousness and reflexes, belonging to the somatic nerves, and when excited, they can cause contraction of the external sphincter, preventing voiding [16]. The sensory nerves of the bladder contain two types of nerve fibers: pain fibers and proprioceptive fibers. Pain fibers mainly receive stimuli from excessive stretching of the bladder wall, stones, inflammation, and malignant tumors through the parasympathetic nerves, causing lower abdominal pain, while proprioception mainly transmits the urge to urinate caused by urine expansion. Figure 2.3 is from Weledji et al., published in 2019. The diagram of lower urinary tract control nerves is shown in "The Anatomy of Voiding: What Every Physician Should Know" [5].

2.2.4 Physiological Function of the Bladder

The bladder is an organ for urine storage and excretion. The storage and excretion of urine in a normal bladder are mainly carried out through

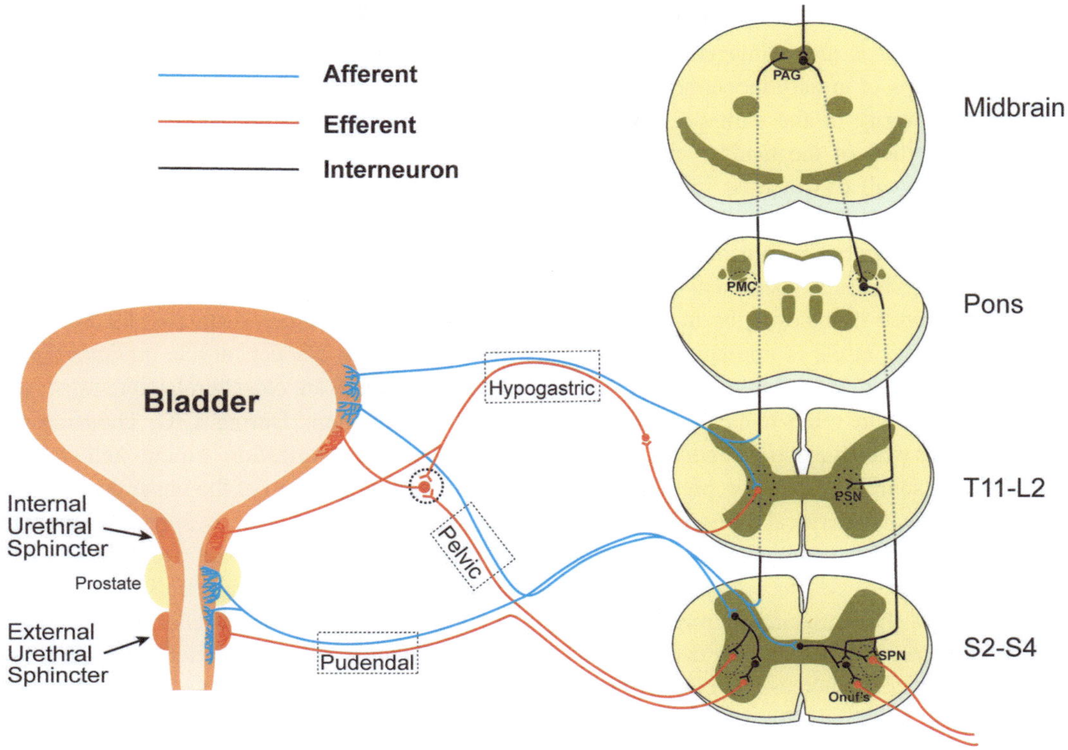

Abbreviation: PAG, periaqueductal grey; PMC, pontine micturition center;
PSN, Propriospinal neuron; Onuf's, Onuf's nucleus; SPN, sacral parasympa thetic nucleus

Fig. 2.3 Nerve distribution of normal lower urinary tract control

peripheral nerve pathways, namely, the sacral parasympathetic nerves (pelvic nerves), the thoracolumbar sympathetic nerves (inferior abdominal nerves and sympathetic trunk), and the sacral somatic nerves (mainly the pudendal nerves) [5]. The detrusor and the internal sphincter of the bladder are dually innervated by the parasympathetic and sympathetic nerves. The acetylcholine released by the postganglionic neurons of the parasympathetic nerves can stimulate the detrusor M-type cholinergic receptors, causing the detrusor to contract and the internal sphincter to relax, thereby promoting voiding. The urine continuously produced by the kidneys is stored in the bladder through the peristalsis of the ureters. When the bladder is full, the stretch receptors in the bladder wall are pulled, and the voiding reflex lower center in the sacral segment of the spinal cord is reached through the afferent nerve fibers, and voiding is controlled by the parasympathetic nerves. For normal adults, when the bladder filling information reaches the brain, voiding can be controlled through subjective sensation. The diaphragm and abdominal muscles can increase the pressure in the bladder during voiding, which has an auxiliary effect on urine excretion [17].

The control of urine in normal males relies on the following two parts: (1) The proximal urethral sphincter includes the bladder neck and the prostatic urethra above the verumontanum. (2) The distal urethral sphincter can be divided into two parts: the posterior urethra below the verumontanum and the external urethral sphincter.

Regardless of males or females, the bladder neck (the urethral smooth muscle controlled by the sympathetic nerves) is the main force to stop the outflow of urine. In males, if the function of the proximal urethral sphincter is completely lost (such as after prostate hyperplasia surgery) and the distal urethral sphincter is intact, voiding can still be controlled as usual. If the function of the distal urethral sphincter is also damaged, it can cause different degrees of urinary incontinence depending on the severity of the damage. In females, when the function of the bladder neck is completely lost, it will cause stress urinary incontinence. When the function of the external urethral sphincter controlled by the somatic nerves (pudendal nerves) is completely lost, it will not cause urinary incontinence in males if the function of the urethral smooth muscle is normal; in females, it can cause stress urinary incontinence [18].

Detrusor pressure refers to the pressure exerted on the bladder when the detrusor contracts, which is the main source of bladder pressure during voiding and the most critical driving force for initiating voiding. Urodynamic study (UDS) could dynamically record detrusor pressure to reflect the function of the detrusor. The maximum pressure of the detrusor in children decreases with age, resulting in an increase in bladder compliance. Normal children's detrusor is mainly controlled by the nervous system. The impulses from the nervous system reach the neuromuscular junction, where electrical signals are converted into mechanical signals, causing the bladder muscle to contract and the pressure inside the bladder to rise. At the same time, the urethral sphincter opens, urine is expelled, and a certain speed is produced, i.e., the urine flow rate. The bladder muscle can also produce a type of non-inhibitory contraction. In normal children, non-inhibitory contractions of the bladder muscle generally occur within the age of 8. Under pathological conditions, such as central nervous system maldevelopment or disease, urinary tract infection, etc., the occurrence rate of non-inhibitory contractions of the bladder muscle can increase. Non-inhibitory contractions of the bladder muscle in children manifest as frequent voiding, urgency, incontinence, and enuresis. The bladder capacity increases with age, and the average bladder capacity of adults is 350–500 mL [10].

The maximum capacity of the bladder is 800 mL, the bladder capacity of a newborn is about one-tenth of that of an adult, the capacity of females is less than that of males, and the capacity of the elderly increases due to low bladder muscle tension. High bladder pressure, decreased compliance, and bladder muscle-sphincter dyssynergia are high-risk factors for upper urinary tract damage. In children with urinary disorders caused by NB and other conditions, factors such as bladder wall thickening, bladder interstitial fibrosis, and nerve lesions cause a significant decrease in bladder compliance, leading to an increase in bladder muscle pressure during the filling phase, resulting in VUR [19]. Therefore, decreased bladder compliance and high bladder muscle pressure during the storage phase are closely related to upper urinary tract dilation. During CIC, choosing the appropriate catheterization timing and volume can protect the function of the upper urinary tract and prevent diseases such as upper urinary tract dilation, hydronephrosis, and even uremia. The bladder capacity of patients of different ages is different. Children have a smaller bladder capacity and require shorter catheterization intervals and relatively smaller catheterization volumes, while the elderly have a larger bladder capacity and require relatively longer catheterization intervals and larger catheterization volumes.

In summary, we have introduced the anatomy and physiological diseases of the urethra and bladder related to CIC. Understanding these knowledge, for patients to perform CIC themselves, as well as family members and caregivers to help patients catheterize, has great reference and guidance significance. Familiarity with the anatomical features of the urethra is the basis for completing CIC. Understanding the anatomy and pathophysiology of the urinary system can help us understand why we need to perform CIC.

References

1. Bai S, Ying D. Systematic anatomy [M]. 8th ed. Beijing: People's Medical Publishing House; 2013.
2. Mahadevan V. Anatomy of the lower urinary tract [J]. Surgery (Oxford). 2019;37(7):351–8.
3. Du X, Su Z. Progress in the study of female urinary control related functional anatomy [J]. Chin Med Eng. 2009;17(5):346–54. [都兴华，苏泽轩. 女性控尿相关功能解剖的研究进展. 中国医学工程，2009;17(5):346–54].
4. Yucel S, Baskin LS. An anatomical description of the male and female urethral sphincter complex [J]. J Urol.

2004;171(5):1890–7. https://doi.org/10.1097/01.ju.0000124106.16505.df.
5. Weledji EP, Eyongeta D, Ngounou E. The anatomy of urination: what every physician should know [J]. Clin Anat. 2019;32(1):60–7. https://doi.org/10.1002/ca.23296.
6. De Groat WC, Griffiths D, Yoshimura N. Neural control of the lower urinary tract [J]. Compr Physiol. 2015;5(1):327–96. https://doi.org/10.1002/cphy.c130056.
7. Sampselle CM, Delancey JO. Anatomy of female continence [J]. J Wound Ostomy Continence Nurs. 1998;25(2):63–70, 72–4. https://doi.org/10.1016/s1071-5754(98)90091-2.
8. Yang X, Wang X, Gao Z, et al. The anatomical pathogenesis of stress urinary incontinence in women [J]. Medicina (Kaunas). 2022;59(1):5. https://doi.org/10.3390/medicina59010005.
9. Schimpf MO, Rahn DD, Wheeler TL, et al. Sling surgery for stress urinary incontinence in women: a systematic review and metaanalysis [J]. Am J Obstet Gynecol. 2014;211(1):71.e1–71.e27. https://doi.org/10.1016/j.ajog.2014.01.030.
10. Robson WL, Leung AK, Thomason MA. Catheterization of the bladder in infants and children [J]. Clin Pediatr (Phila). 2006;45(9):795–800. https://doi.org/10.1177/0009922806295277.
11. Bogart LM, Berry SH, Clemens JQ. Symptoms of interstitial cystitis, painful bladder syndrome and similar diseases in women: a systematic review [J]. J Urol. 2007;177(2):450–6. https://doi.org/10.1016/j.juro.2006.09.032.
12. Beauchemin L, Newman DK, Le Danseur M, et al. Best practices for clean intermittent catheterization [J]. Nursing. 2018;48(9):49–54. https://doi.org/10.1097/01.NURSE.0000544216.23783.bc.
13. Aaron L, Franco OE, Hayward SW. Review of prostate anatomy and embryology and the etiology of benign prostatic hyperplasia [J]. Urol Clin North Am. 2016;43(3):279–88. https://doi.org/10.1016/j.ucl.2016.04.012.
14. Fry CH, Vahabi B. The role of the mucosa in normal and abnormal bladder function [J]. Basic Clin Pharmacol Toxicol. 2016;119(Suppl 3):57–62. https://doi.org/10.1111/bcpt.12626.
15. Drake MJ. The integrative physiology of the bladder [J]. Ann R Coll Surg Engl. 2007;89(6):580–5. https://doi.org/10.1308/003588407x205585.
16. Beckel JM, Holstege G. Neuroanatomy of the lower urinary tract [J]. Handb Exp Pharmacol. 2011;202:99–116. https://doi.org/10.1007/978-3-642-16499-6_6.
17. De Groat WC, Yoshimura N. Anatomy and physiology of the lower urinary tract [J]. Handb Clin Neurol. 2015;130:61–108. https://doi.org/10.1016/b978-0-444-63247-0.00005-5.
18. Shah AP, Mevcha A, Wilby D, et al. Continence and micturition: an anatomical basis [J]. Clin Anat. 2014;27(8):1275–83. https://doi.org/10.1002/ca.22388.
19. Wang QW, Wen JG, Song DK, et al. Is it possible to use urodynamic variables to predict upper urinary tract dilatation in children with neurogenic bladder-sphincter dysfunction? [J]. BJU Int. 2006;98(6):1295–300. https://doi.org/10.1111/j.1464-410X.2006.06402.x.

3 Choosing the Right Catheter and Related Consumables Is a Condition for Successful CIC

Jian-Guo Wen

In recent years, the application of CIC and CISC has gradually become widespread. It is now recognized that CIC can effectively reduce the risk of infection, reduce complications, and improve quality of life, and the procedure is simple [1]. However, the smooth progress of CIC cannot be separated from the correct selection of related catheters and consumables and professional procedure skills [2, 3]. The following focuses on how to choose the various catheters and basic consumables needed for CIC.

The so-called catheters and consumables are the consumable accessories used in the process of CIC such as the consumables that need to be prepared before the procedure (commonly needed in hospital procedures, clean disposable gloves can be used at home or in the work environment, or no gloves are needed, just washing hands), disinfection supplies during the procedure (disposable wet wipes or cleaners and towels, disinfectant sprays or disinfectant cotton pads, sterile gauze), types of catheters (uncoated catheters, coated catheters, closed system catheters), catheter materials (PVC, silicone, rubber, latex), catheter models, catheter tip shapes (straight, curved head), various lubricants (if it is not a hydrophilic catheter, water-soluble lubricants, paraffin oil, and lidocaine gel are needed), auxiliary CIC devices such as mirrors (commonly used in female catheterization; those with magnifying effects are better), toilets, or urine collection containers and storage bags. In order to correctly perform CIC procedures and achieve satisfactory therapeutic effects, it is necessary to understand the models, sizes, materials, functions, and roles of these consumables and supplies [4].

CIC and CISC are currently the preferred methods for treating NB [5]. The efficacy depends on the operation technique, including the type of catheter and lubricant used, the handling and insertion method of the catheter, etc. During the procedure, choosing the appropriate catheter can reduce the incidence of complications. With the continuous emergence of new technologies and new materials, the catheter is also updated in terms of material and design, and there are many types of catheters on the market. When patients choose a catheter, they need to consider their own conditions comprehensively, such as the possible degree of damage to the urethra, hand function, vision, urethral sensitivity, gender, age, economic conditions, etc. Cleaning gloves, wipes as well as essential consumables such as cleaning towels, gauze, cotton pads, mirrors, urine collectors and disinfectant spray, are also needed during the procedure [6–8].

J.-G. Wen (✉)
Pediatric Urodynamic Center/Department of Urology, First Affiliated Hospital of Zhengzhou University, Zhengzhou, China

J.-G. Wen (ed.), *Progress in Clean Intermittent Catheterization*, Experts' Perspectives on Medical Advances, https://doi.org/10.1007/978-981-97-5021-4_3

3.1 Procedural Prerequisites

Maintaining hand hygiene is a prerequisite for performing CIC. Consumables required for hand hygiene include clean towels or paper towels, soap or liquid soap for hand washing, clean water, etc. However, no hand washing method can completely eliminate bacteria deep in the skin. If conditions permit, sterile gloves or relatively clean disposable gloves can be prepared [8].

3.2 Disinfectants

Disinfection is an important means to kill pathogenic microorganisms and thus prevent infection. Standard disinfection procedures before catheterization can effectively prevent and reduce the occurrence of urinary tract infections [9, 10].

The disinfection procedure during the CIC process mainly involves the urethral orifice and nearby skin, mainly involving the urethral mucosa. Disinfectants usually include disinfectant cotton balls, disinfectant cotton pads, and disinfectant cotton swabs. Disinfectant cotton balls generally need to be operated with tweezers and are used more in hospitals. Cotton pads or cotton swabs are commonly used at home and can be chosen according to the user's operating habits. The choice of disinfectants mainly involves the choice of disinfectant. Among commonly used disinfectants, povidone-iodine and benzalkonium bromide are suitable for mucosal disinfection. Povidone-iodine is not as effective as iodine alcohol in killing bacteria, but it can be used for skin and mucosal disinfection and can also treat burns, trichomonas vaginitis, fungal vaginitis, skin fungal infections, etc. Burns, frostbite, knife wounds, abrasions, and other general traumas can be effectively disinfected with povidone-iodine, which is less irritating and less painful than iodine alcohol and alcohol. Povidone-iodine can be directly applied for skin disinfection treatment; diluted twice for oral inflammation gargling; and diluted ten times for vaginal inflammation washing treatment. Benzalkonium bromide is a quaternary ammonium salt cationic surfactant with broad-spectrum bactericidal properties, strong and fast bactericidal action, low toxicity, no irritation to skin and tissues, strong penetration, and no corrosive effect on metal and rubber products. Benzalkonium bromide can kill various Gram-positive and Gram-negative bacteria such as staphylococci, typhoid bacilli, paratyphoid bacilli, *E. coli*, and tuberculosis, fungi, etc. It can be used for surgical disinfection, skin disinfection, mucosal disinfection, purulent skin treatment, etc. Therefore, these two disinfectants are the preferred choices for catheterization procedures, and sterile gauze or sterile cotton swabs are also indispensable disposable items for disinfection. Patients can choose clean towels and warm water to clean the perineal area according to their own economic conditions or use disposable wet wipes for disinfection before catheterization [8].

3.3 Catheter

During CIC, choosing the appropriate catheter can reduce the incidence of complications. With the emergence of new technologies and materials, catheters are also updated in terms of material and design, and there are many types of catheters on the market. When patients choose a catheter, they need to consider their own conditions comprehensively, such as the degree of injury, hand function, degree of visual impairment, urethral sensitivity, gender, age, and economic conditions [11–13]. The 2011 version of the "Neurogenic Bladder Care Guidelines" proposes that the ideal catheter for CIC should meet the following conditions [14]: (1) sterile; (2) good biocompatibility; (3) soft and easy to bend; (4) made of high shape-retaining materials; (5) non-traumatic; (6) ready to use. When patients choose a catheter, they can use the above conditions as basic consideration standards, which ensure the safety and ease of use of the catheter [12]. Considering the specific catheter application, we can also discuss the selection skills of the catheter from the following perspectives.

3.3.1 Types of Catheters

The common catheters currently include uncoated catheters, coated catheters, and closed system catheters [4]. Uncoated catheters, also known as ordinary catheters, are commonly used for CIC and are recommended to be lubricated when used. Uncoated catheters are mostly disposable, and some can be reused. Reusable catheters are usually made of materials such as silicone, latex, fiberglass, and stainless steel. There are certain disadvantages to choosing this type of catheter. Long-term use cannot guarantee the cleanliness and storage effect of the catheter, so it is not recommended to reuse this type of catheter. Krassioukov and others conducted a survey on the utilization rate of catheterization and the frequency of UTIs at the 2012 London Paralympics and the 2013 World Cycling Championships. Participants (n = 61) were divided into developing and developed countries according to their economic conditions. Participants shared their current catheterization methods. Patients from developing countries had a much higher rate of catheter reuse, and the number of urinary tract infections per year was twice that of patients who did not reuse catheters. Coated catheters have a gel surface or are wrapped in gel. These catheters can be used for CIC and sterile CIC techniques. They are designed for one-time use, pre-coated for easy insertion and removal, thereby reducing the risk of urethral mucosal irritation, which is more common in uncoated products. Catheters have two types of coatings, antibiotic and hydrophilic, and cannot be reused. The antibiotic coating may have a local antibacterial effect, and some antibiotic-coated catheters also have a hydrophilic coating. The problem with this type of catheter is that patients may be allergic to the antibiotic coating and there is a possibility of secondary infection, and it can only be used once, so it has not been popularized. Hydrophilic-coated catheters are throughout the entire PVC. The catheter is wrapped in a hydrophilic polymer, mainly polyvinylpyrrolidone (PVP). This increases the hydrophilic lubricity of the catheter surface. When it comes into contact with water, it quickly forms a lubricating film on its surface that is not easy to fall off. During clinical catheterization, this thick, smooth structure on the surface of the catheter ensures that the catheter remains lubricated during insertion and removal, thereby reducing the friction between the catheter and the urethral mucosa. Experiments have shown that its lubrication degree is 10–100 times that of ordinary catheter products. It is a safe substance that does not cause allergies in the human body, so this type of catheter is also called a super smooth catheter (Fig. 3.1), especially recommended for pediatric patients [15]. The advantages of the super smooth catheter are as follows: First, it has super strong lubricity and biocompatibility. The tube body is fully lubricated, and the lubrication is sufficient, which can ensure the reduction of uneven smearing when manually applying lubricant, reduce the irritation to the urethral mucosa, reduce the probability of damage to the urethral epithelial tissue, alleviate the patient's lower limb nerve pain and discomfort, relieve the patient's tension and anxiety, make the patient feel comfortable, and also reduce the probability of external factors inducing the patient's nerve pain. Because the lubrication effect is long-lasting, during the entire catheterization process, the chance of urethral stimulation and spasm is reduced, and the success rate of catheterization is much higher than that of ordinary catheters. The second is the convenience of use. Before catheterization, just immerse the super smooth catheter in sterile saline for a few seconds to achieve a fully lubricated effect. The procedure is convenient. A newly launched super

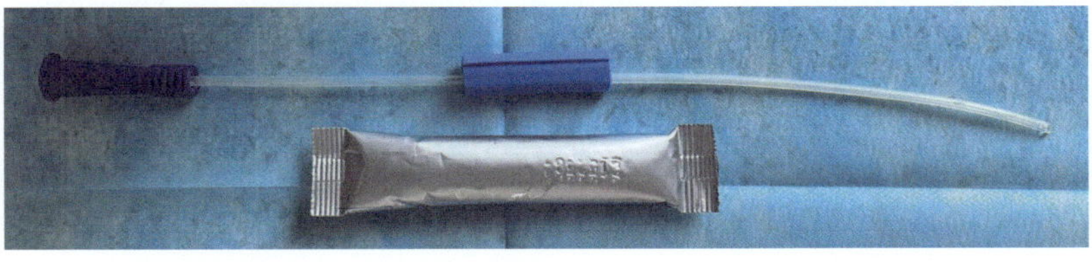

Fig. 3.1 Super smooth catheter

smooth catheter with its own sterile water bag has better convenience. When using it, just squeeze the water bag in the single package to let the sterile water flow out and wet the tube body, which can conveniently activate the hydrophilic coating, especially convenient when carrying out. At the same time, the use of its own sterile water can also eliminate the possibility of contaminating the catheter with other water sources, reducing the risk of urinary tract infections. Finally, it can reduce the incidence of urinary tract infections. The front end of the catheter increases the discharge hole, which can completely clear the post-voided residual (PVR). The tube body is transparent, and the color and nature of the urine can be observed during the catheterization process, and abnormalities in the urine (such as color, transparency, presence or absence of precipitated flocculent matter, etc.) can be found in time, thereby reducing the bacterial risk of the urinary system and the possibility of urinary tract infections. The catheterization process is simple, and the texture is slightly hard, so that the patient can master the procedure after discharge.

Closed catheter system catheter: This type of catheter has a lubricating oil or hydrophilic coating or antibacterial coating on the surface, and the catheter is directly connected to the urine collection bag. Some spinal cord injury (SCI) patients are suitable for using this type of catheter. Most closed catheter systems are designed with an introducer tip about 15 mm long to prevent the catheter from being contaminated and bringing bacteria into the bladder. During catheterization, the operator cannot touch the catheter directly with their hands, so there are certain requirements for hand function [16–18].

3.3.2 Material of the Catheter

Different materials of catheters stimulate the urethral mucosa differently. The materials of catheters used for intermittent catheterization are diverse, some contain latex, and some do not. Non-latex catheters are currently the most commonly used, and the material is medical-grade plastic, such as polyvinyl chloride (PVC) or silicone. Silicone catheters and PVC catheters have better biocompatibility, less cytotoxicity, various hardness levels, a wide range of diameters, and a harder head end, which facilitates smooth insertion. The catheter wall is soft, reducing the incidence of infection and alleviating irritation to the urinary tract (Fig. 3.2) [19, 20].

PVC is a thermoplastic polymer, and the polymerization methods mainly include suspension polymerization, emulsion polymerization, and bulk polymerization. Its advantages in the medical field are transparency, flexibility, reliability, durability, easy sterilization, compatibility, resistance to chemical stress cracking, and easy processing.

Recyclable, cheap PVC is widely used in medical products, such as blood bags, pipes, disposable examination gloves, and medical trays. Sallami and others believe that patients tolerate PVC catheters the best, and PVC is also relatively cheap, widely used at home and abroad [16].

Siliconized latex catheters and plastic catheters have medium toxicity. Because their surfaces are siliconized, they are not easy to form bacterial biofilms. The catheter is durable and highly flexible, which can effectively help bladder drainage, so urinary complications are less. Silicone has many unique properties, such as good physiological inertia, resistance to body fluid corrosion, aging resistance under harsh environmental conditions, excellent biocompatibility, minimal inflammatory response to human tissues, no foreign body reaction in the body, and no inflammatory reaction to surrounding tissues, so it is widely used in the medical field.

Rubber, especially white rubber catheters, has a high level of toxicity, causing the most obvious urethral damage, which can cause complete destruction of the urethral epithelium, significant infiltration of inflammatory cells, exudation, and bleeding. Red rubber catheters contain latex components and are not suitable for patients allergic to latex. This type of catheter is softer and more difficult to insert [21].

The additives added to latex migrate from the inside to the surface, easily stimulating the urethra to produce white secretions, causing the patient to have an inflammatory reaction.

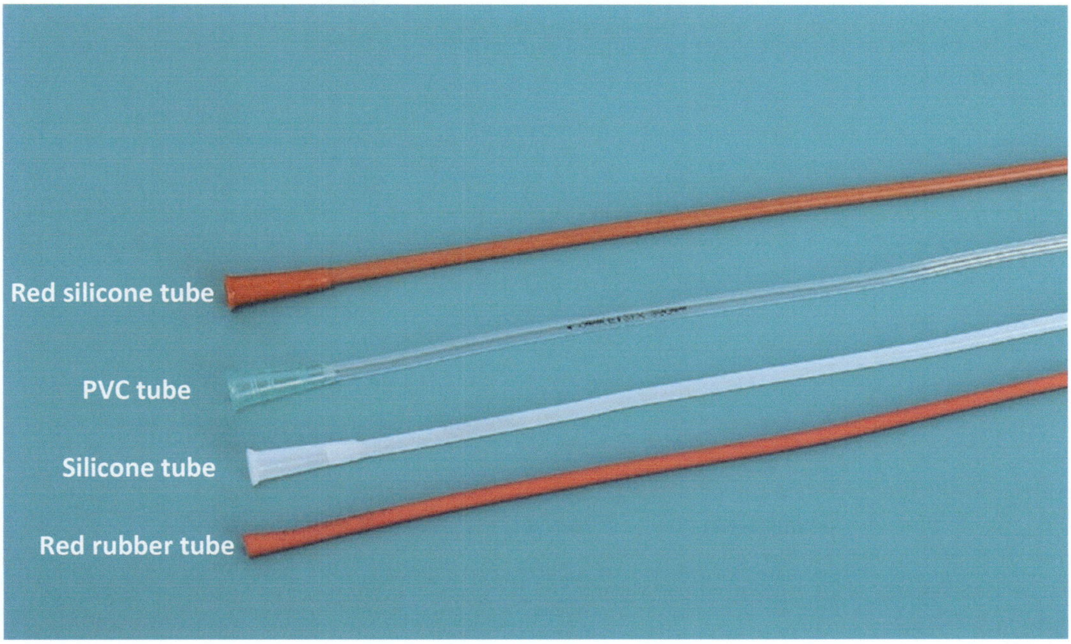

Fig. 3.2 Catheters of various materials (see color insert 1 for color images)

3.3.3 Size of the Catheter

The catheters used for CIC come in seven common sizes from 6 to 18 Fr. Sizes 6–12 Fr are suitable for children, and sizes 10–16 Fr are suitable for adults (10–14 Fr for males, 14–16 Fr for females). Due to different anatomical structures, patients of different genders can choose catheters of different lengths as needed. Adult male can choose 12 inches (about 40 cm) in length. Women and children generally do not need a catheter longer than 6 inches (about 20 cm) due to their shorter urethra. Shorter catheters are less likely to coil and knot, facilitating urine discharge and patient self-procedure. Of course, different application scenarios will have different requirements for catheter length, and the appropriate size should be chosen according to the actual situation. If you are unsure of the size, always start with a smaller size, and then increase the diameter as needed. There are a variety of lengths to choose from; please use the appropriate length according to the patient's needs. See Tables 3.1 and 3.2 for the model and corresponding catheter diameter of children's catheters.

Table 3.1 Children's CIC age and corresponding catheter size

Age (year)	Size (Fr)
0~2	6
2~5	6/8
5~10	8/10
10~16	10/12
16+	12/16

Table 3.2 International catheter model and tube diameter parameter comparison table

Catheter size (Fr)	Catheter outer diameter (mm)	Corresponding connector color
6	2.0	Grass green
8	2.7	Light blue
10	3.3	Black
12	4.0	White
14	4.7	Green
16	5.3	Orange
18	6.0	Red

3.3.4 Shape of the Catheter Tip

The tip of the catheter can be made into different types, commonly straight and curved. (1) Straight catheter: Suitable for male, female, and child

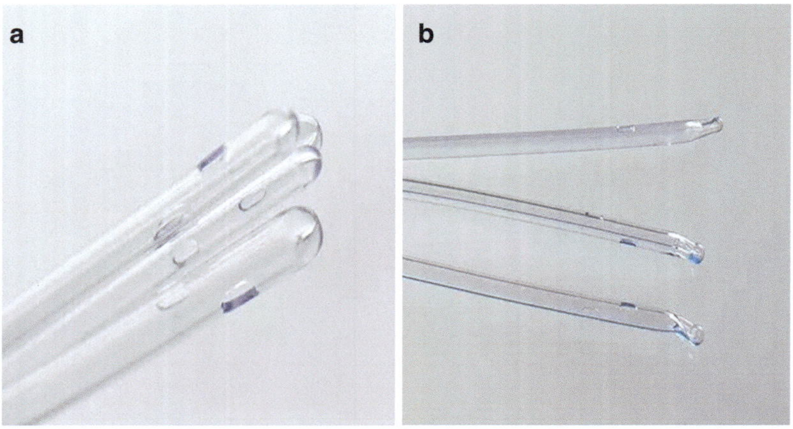

Fig. 3.3 Straight (**a**), curved (**b**) catheter (see color insert 2 for color image)

patients, urine flows into the catheter lumen from the two drainage openings of the catheter (Fig. 3.3). (2) Curved catheter: The tip is designed to be arc-shaped, with one to three drainage openings.

The slanted tip of the catheter provides directional stability, and the tip is slightly harder than the standard model, making it easier to insert into the blocked area. Therefore, this type of catheter can pass through the urethral membrane and prostate of patients related to prostate hyperplasia or narrowing or scar formation. For male patients (adults or children) with special indications (such as enlarged prostate), this curved catheter is the preferred choice (Fig. 3.3b).

3.3.5 Drainage Hole and Smoothness of the Tube Body

Catheterization is an invasive procedure; a rough catheter will directly damage the urethral mucosa; therefore, when choosing a catheter, one must choose a tube with a sufficiently smooth body and drainage opening [22]. Generally speaking, drainage holes made with hot melt technology are smoother than cold punched holes.

3.3.6 Catheter Length

According to anatomical standards, the length of adult male urethra is 17–20 cm, and the length of the female urethra is 3–5 cm. In view of this, the internationally common catheter length is classified as three types: 40 cm for adult males, 15 ~ 20 cm for adult females, and 25 cm for children. In the actual procedure, different catheterization scenarios require different lengths of catheters. For example, in bed catheterization, if the catheter is too short, it can easily cause inconvenience in urine collection and is more likely to dirty the bed, so choosing a longer catheter is more appropriate; some patients catheterize while sitting on the toilet; if the catheter is too long, it is not convenient to drain urine into the toilet, so a shorter catheter should be chosen at this time [23].

3.3.7 Advantages of Disposable Catheters in China

The disposable catheter produced in China is mainly composed of a catheter and a connector; it is a non-balloon single-lumen type, made of soft polyvinyl chloride plastic, sterilized by ethylene oxide, and for single use. Its advantages are the following: (1) The safety of the catheter material to the body has been clinically proven over a long period of time, it can be used with confidence, and the independent sterilization packaging can also maintain the sterility of the product well. (2) The disposable catheter is discarded after use, making it more convenient to use, without worrying about the effectiveness of cleaning and disinfection. (3) Except for the slightly higher price of the catheter with a hydrophilic coating, ordinary catheters are quite economical and affordable, with good quality catheters costing more than 1 yuan each, and one is used for each catheterization. Reusable catheters are more expensive due to the high cost of silicone, and the lifespan of the catheter may be reduced due to some factors in actual procedure. If calculated based on the routine intermittent catheterization four to six times a day, the economic expenditure of disposable catheters is not much different from that of reusable catheters, and the economy of the two types of catheters is similar. If the patient can excrete part of the urine on their own and the number of daily intermittent catheterizations is less, disposable catheters are more economical than reusable catheters [1, 24, 25].

3.4 Catheter Lubricant

The female urethra is shorter, and the physiological structure is relatively simple; some women can complete catheterization smoothly without using a lubricant. The male urethra is longer, and the physiological structure is more complex, complications are more likely to occur, and the lubrication of the catheter is very important, directly affecting the difficulty of inserting the catheter, which is a widely concerned issue when performing CIC. In 2011, the "Neurogenic Bladder Care Guidelines" launched by the Rehabilitation Nursing Professional Committee of the China Rehabilitation Medical Association clearly pointed out: For non-coated or ordinary catheters, a lubricant must be used. Using a lubricant can reduce the friction between the catheter and the urethral mucosa, provide comfort, and allow the catheter to be smoothly inserted into the bladder.

For a long time, there have been many types of catheter lubricants, and gel, water solvent or edible oil, liquid paraffin, or even clear water are chosen according to economic conditions. Lidocaine gel is considered to effectively reduce the occurrence of complications such as urethral bleeding. The most commonly used in clinical practice are paraffin oil and water-soluble lubricants. So, which is more suitable for CIC, paraffin oil or water-soluble lubricant? In recent years, many professionals have conducted research on this, and it is generally believed that water-soluble lubricants are superior to paraffin oil. We can understand this from the following aspects.

1. Paraffin oil, also known as mineral oil, is a colorless and odorless mixture obtained from the distillation of crude oil. Data shows that poorly refined mineral oil with many impurities has a certain carcinogenicity. Since paraffin oil is extracted from petroleum, it is a colorless, transparent, and odorless viscous liquid. If it is not well refined and the impurity content is too high, it may cause cancer or other harm to the human body. Therefore, the use of paraffin oil carries certain potential risks.

   Paraffin oil belongs to petroleum-based lubricants and has a significant corrosive effect on natural latex products. If the user's catheter is made of latex material, it should not use paraffin oil for lubrication. Studies have shown that when paraffin oil is used to lubricate surgical instruments, scattered milky white spots often appear on the cleaned instruments and turntables, forming a new source of pollution. This phenomenon does not occur when water-soluble lubricants are used. Paraffin oil is insoluble in water and easily adheres. When used as a lubricant in routine catheterization procedures, although it can play a certain lubricating role, it has disadvantages such as not being easily absorbed by the body, not easy to excrete, and easy to adhere to the urethra. CIC often needs to be persisted for a long time, even for life. Long-term residual paraffin oil in the body can easily cause complications such as urethral stricture and urinary tract infection.

2. The main ingredients of water-soluble lubricants are pure water and fiber, as well as glycerin, propylene glycol, fragrance, trichlorosucrose, etc., which are easily absorbed by the body and have no toxic side effects. The lubrication effect is good, it feels refreshing and not greasy when used, and it will not remain in the body for a long time. Its biocompatibility is better than that of paraffin oil [15].

   Therefore, when patients perform CIC, it is recommended to use water-soluble lubricants to lubricate the catheter. Paraffin oil may harm health, and its lubrication effect is not ideal, so it should be avoided as much as possible.

3.5 Common Self-Adaptive Auxiliary Devices Used in CIC

Common self-adaptive auxiliary devices in the female CIC process include Betty hooks (to assist in pulling down pants/underwear), leg spreaders (mainly used for female patients who need it due to leg spasms), catheter racks (to assist in catheter fixation), and labia spreaders (to assist in expanding the labia and maintaining fixation), vaginal introducers (easier to identify the vaginal and urethral orifice), and mirrors (magnifying mirrors are better, used to identify the vaginal and urethral orifice).

In the male CIC process, commonly used auxiliary devices include Betty hooks, leg spreaders, catheter racks, and penis collars (to assist in exposing and fixing the penis) (Fig. 3.4).

Common self-assist devices used in the process of children's clean catheterization include flat bed surfaces or tables, and infants require changing tables, etc. Special teaching aids for pediatrics also need to be provided, including training dolls, coloring books, flashcards, books, games, videos, etc., to alleviate the discomfort of children during the catheterization process [23].

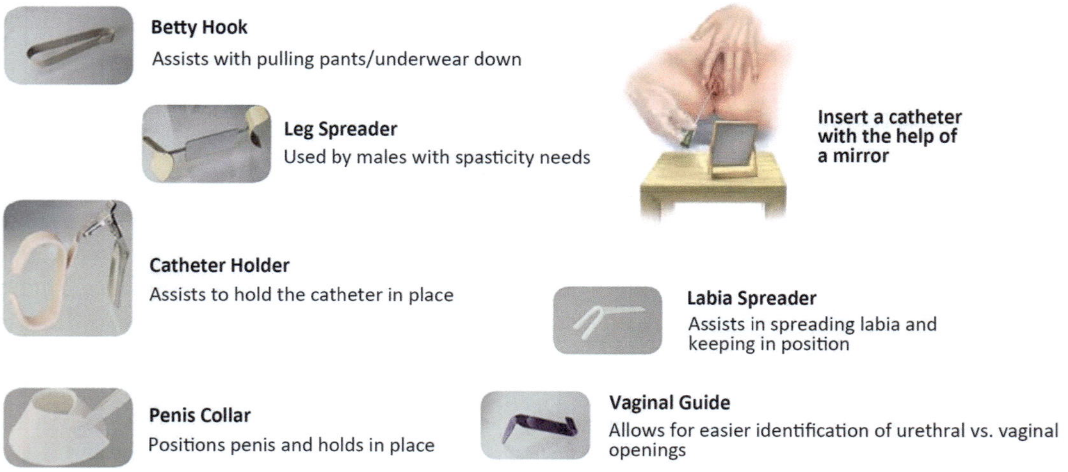

Fig. 3.4 Self-adaptive CIC assistive device (see color insert 3 for color image)

3.6 Urine Collector

During the CIC process, for children or patients with special needs, after inserting the catheter into the bladder through the urethra, the urine is led out to a graduated cup or a graduated urinal. If in school, outdoor activity areas, shopping malls, etc., the urine can be directly discharged into the toilet [26].

In summary, the catheters and consumables used for CIC can basically meet the needs of current patients, but some consumables still need to be improved, such as the material and type of the catheter. When patients choose catheters and consumables, they need to consider their own conditions comprehensively, such as newborns and infants, who should choose small catheters as much as possible, and female patients should choose shorter catheters. In addition, patients need to have a clear concept of the use of catheters and need to receive professional medical staff training and guidance before use. For patients with poor economic conditions, especially female patients, they can buy cheaper domestic catheters and achieve good results, but it is not recommended to reuse catheters. Choosing the right catheter and consumables can both improve the quality of life of patients and reduce the incidence of urinary system infections.

References

1. Zhao CC, Comiter CV, Elliott CS. Single-use catheters: evidence and environmental impact [J]. BJU Int. 2024;133(6):638–45. https://doi.org/10.1111/bju.16313.
2. Elliott CS. Sustainability in urology: single-use versus reusable catheters for intermittent catheterization [J]. Eur Urol Focus. 2023;9(6):888–90. https://doi.org/10.1016/j.euf.2023.09.012.
3. Ye D, Chen Y, Jian Z, et al. Catheters for intermittent catheterization: a systematic review and network meta-analysis [J]. Spinal Cord. 2021;59(6):587–95. https://doi.org/10.1038/s41393-021-00620-w.
4. Goetz LI, Droste L, Klausner AP, Al E. Catheters used for intermittent catheterization. In: Newman DK, Rovner ES, Wein AJ, et al., editors. Clinical application of urologic catheters and products [M]. Cham: Springer International Publishing; 2018.
5. Corcos J. Evaluation and treatment of neurogenic bladder [M]. Beijing: People's Medical Publishing House; 2010.
6. Avery M, Prieto J, Okamoto I, et al. Reuse of intermittent catheters: a qualitative study of IC users' perspectives [J]. BMJ Open. 2018;8(8):e021554. https://doi.org/10.1136/bmjopen-2018-021554.
7. Mcclurg D, Coyle J, Long A, et al. A two phased study on health care professionals' perceptions of single or multi-use of intermittent catheters [J]. Int J Nurs Stud. 2017;72:83–90. https://doi.org/10.1016/j.ijnurstu.2017.04.009.
8. Clinical Advisory Board for Intermittent Catheterization. Clean intermittent catheterization: guidelines for healthcare professionals [J/OL]. 2013.
9. Takahashi R, Sekido N, Matsuoka M, et al. Hygiene management of intermittent self-catheterization using reusable silicone catheters in people with spinal cord lesions: a cross-sectional Internet survey in Japan [J]. Low Urin Tract Symptoms. 2023;15(5):165–72. https://doi.org/10.1111/luts.12490.
10. Sekiguchi Y, Yao Y, Ohko Y, et al. Self-sterilizing catheters with titanium dioxide photocatalyst thin films for clean intermittent catheterization: basis and study of clinical use [J]. Int J Urol. 2007;14(5):426–30. https://doi.org/10.1111/j.1442-2042.2007.01743.x.
11. Grasdal M, Walter M, Krassioukov AV. The microbiological and physical properties of catheters for intermittent catheterization: a systematic review on the impact of reuse and cleaning [J]. Spinal Cord. 2022;60(7):581–93. https://doi.org/10.1038/s41393-021-00740-3.
12. Fang H, Lin J, Liang L, et al. A nonsurgical and nonpharmacological care bundle for preventing upper urinary tract damage in patients with spinal cord injury and neurogenic bladder [J]. Int J Nurs Pract. 2020;26(2):e12761. https://doi.org/10.1111/ijn.12761.
13. Håkansson M. Reuse versus single-use catheters for intermittent catheterization: what is safe and preferred? Review of current status [J]. Spinal Cord. 2014;52(7):511–6. https://doi.org/10.1038/sc.2014.79.
14. Gomelsky A, Lemack GE, Castano Botero JC, et al. Current and future international patterns of care of neurogenic bladder after spinal cord injury [J]. World J Urol. 2018;36(10):1613–9. https://doi.org/10.1007/s00345-018-2277-8.
15. Place J. Advances in clean intermittent self-catheterisation: impact on trauma and urinary tract infections [J]. Br J Nurs. 2023;32(Sup18):S5–7. https://doi.org/10.12968/bjon.2023.32.Sup18.S5.
16. Liang Z. Research progress on intermittent catheterization [J]. Chin J Rehabil Theory Pract. 2013;19(4):360–1. [梁志. 间歇导尿的研究进展. 中国康复理论与实践, 2013;19(4):360–1].
17. Chartier-Kastler E, Denys P. Intermittent catheterization with hydrophilic catheters as a treatment of

chronic neurogenic urinary retention [J]. Neurourol Urodyn. 2011;30(1):21–31. https://doi.org/10.1002/nau.20929.
18. Sarica S, Akkoc Y, Karapolat H, Aktug H. Comparison of the use of conventional, hydrophilic and gel-lubricated catheters with regard to urethral micro trauma, urinary system infection, and patient satisfaction in patients with spinal cord injury: a randomized controlled study [J]. Eur J Phys Rehabil Med. 2010;46(4):473–9.
19. Jackson MJ, Veeratterapillay R, Harding CK, Dorkin TJ. Intermittent self-dilatation for urethral stricture disease in males [J]. Cochrane Database Syst Rev. 2014;2014(12):CD010258. https://doi.org/10.1002/14651858.CD010258.pub2.
20. Kovindha A, Mai WN, Madersbacher H. Reused silicone catheter for clean intermittent catheterization (CIC): is it safe for spinal cord-injured (SCI) men? [J]. Spinal Cord. 2004;42(11):638–42. https://doi.org/10.1038/sj.sc.3101646.
21. Goldberg H, Aharony S, Levy Y, et al. Low prevalence of latex allergy in children with spinal dysraphism in non-latex-free environment [J]. J Pediatr Urol. 2016;12(1):52.e51–5. https://doi.org/10.1016/j.jpurol.2015.07.011.
22. Diokno AC, Mitchell BA, Nash AJ, Kimbrough JA. Patient satisfaction and the LoFric catheter for clean intermittent catheterization [J]. J Urol. 1995;153(2):349–51. https://doi.org/10.1097/00005392-199502000-00015.
23. Walter M, Christison K, Wyndaele JJM, et al. Response to Elliot and Crew response to Christison et al. Intermittent catheterization: the devil is in the details [J]. J Neurotrauma. 2019;36(10):1678–9. https://doi.org/10.1089/neu.2018.6289.
24. Van Doorn T, Berendsen SA, Scheepe JR, Blok BFM. Single use versus reusable catheters in intermittent catheterisation for treatment of urinary retention: a protocol for a multicentre, prospective, randomised controlled, non-inferiority trial (COMPaRE) [J]. BMJ Open. 2022;12(4):e056649. https://doi.org/10.1136/bmjopen-2021-056649.
25. Getliffe K, Fader M, Allen C, et al. Current evidence on intermittent catheterization: sterile single-use catheters or clean reused catheters and the incidence of UTI [J]. J Wound Ostomy Continence Nurs. 2007;34(3):289–96. https://doi.org/10.1097/01.WON.0000270824.37436.f6.
26. Cardenas DD, Mayo ME, Turner LR. Lower urinary changes over time in suprasacral spinal cord injury [J]. Paraplegia. 1995;33(6):326–9. https://doi.org/10.1038/sc.1995.73.

4 CIC Can Be Widely Applied Clinically

Jian-Guo Wen

CIC can effectively solve the problem of safe urine discharge, prevent VUR and kidney damage, prevent complications of bladder emptying disorders (increased PVR and UTI), and reduce symptoms of urinary incontinence, frequency, and urgency, thereby improving quality of life. CIC is commonly used in patients with difficulty urinating and significant increase in PVR and is one of the effective treatments for dysuria, increased PVR, and overflow incontinence [1, 2]. The causes of overflow incontinence are often due to weak detrusor contraction and lack of detrusor reflex, and the etiology may be the damage of nerve that controls the voiding reflex, bladder outlet obstruction (BOO), or the influence of certain drugs. If there is still a large amount of PVR after the obstruction, drugs and other causes are removed, or when the detrusor contraction force is significantly damaged and cannot be recovered, long-term CIC can be considered. CIC is also often used as a treatment for urinary retention after bladder augmentation (or autologous bladder augmentation and intestinal bladder augmentation), which can effectively prevent urinary system infections and protect upper urinary tract function [3, 4]. With a deeper understanding of CIC, total bladder resection plus controllable bladder surgery has become popular and recognized; CIC has also become the best way to empty the bladder for controllable urinary diversion. Therefore, if there is a bladder emptying disorder (increased PVR) and the catheter can be inserted into the bladder through the urethra or bladder outlet, CIC can be implemented. Therefore, CIC has a wide range of clinical application value. However, if CIC is used improperly, there is also a risk of complications such as UTI. Therefore, the indications for CIC need to be strictly mastered [5].

4.1 Indications for CIC

The physiological function of the bladder is to store urine and intermittently empty according to physiological needs. Therefore, bladder dysfunction is accordingly divided into storage dysfunction and emptying dysfunction. Storage dysfunction mainly includes frequency, urgency, and incontinence; emptying dysfunction mainly includes hesitation in voiding, effort in voiding, and incomplete voiding (emptying disorder). CIC is mainly suitable for patients with bladder emptying dysfunction caused by various reasons, the most common of which is NB and others include non-neurogenic NB, post-intestinal bladder augmentation, post-intestinal bladder replacement, and long-term lower urinary tract obstruction leading to weakened detrusor con-

J.-G. Wen (✉)
Pediatric Urodynamic Center/Department of Urology, First Affiliated Hospital of Zhengzhou University, Zhengzhou, China

J.-G. Wen (ed.), *Progress in Clean Intermittent Catheterization*, Experts' Perspectives on Medical Advances, https://doi.org/10.1007/978-981-97-5021-4_4

traction and excessive post-voided residual (VUR). However, the prerequisite for performing CIC is that the patient has a normal urinary bladder control mechanism, no urinary incontinence occurs during the CIC interval, and there is sufficient bladder capacity [children > their expected maximum bladder capacity, i.e., ((age +1) × 30 mL, adults >300 mL)], normal bladder compliance (>20 mL/cmH_2O) or the end pressure of bladder filling <30 cmH_2O can be made through CIC [6–8].

4.1.1 Neurogenic Bladder

The bladder dysfunction caused by nerve lesions that control the bladder is called NB. The nerve lesions that cause NB can be divided into upper motor neuron lesions (such as central nervous system lesions, including stroke, Parkinson's disease, multiple system sclerosis), spinal cord lesions (including spinal sclerosis, cervical and thoracic intervertebral disc diseases, spinal trauma, etc.), and lower motor neuron lesions (such as pelvic nerve injury, peripheral nerve lesions, diabetes, etc.). Adults are often seen in spinal cord injuries, and children are often seen in congenital spinal canal malformations (spina bifida, spinal meningocele, etc.) [9, 10].

For children with NB, the European "Guidelines for the Diagnosis and Treatment of Children and Adolescents with NB" recommends that children with spina bifida can start CIC from birth if the bladder cannot be emptied, which can reduce kidney complications and increase the probability of bladder function recovery in the future. The earlier CIC starts, the higher the acceptance. For children with low or no sphincter activity or no outlet obstruction, if it is confirmed by ultrasound and UDS that there is almost no PVR, CIC is not necessary, but close follow-up is required [9, 11, 12].

In order to initiate voiding or ensure complete emptying of the bladder, it is necessary to develop a corresponding bladder management program, which includes interventions such as drug treatment, timed voiding, indwelling catheter, manual squeezing (Crede maneuver), urinary diversion, CIC, etc. Among them, CIC is one of the most effective and commonly used methods to help bladder emptying in NB patients. By regularly emptying the bladder, it can avoid overfilling of the bladder, reduce the pressure inside the bladder, improve the blood circulation of the bladder wall, and make the bladder mucosa more resistant to bacterial infections [13].

The advantages of CIC over continuous indwelling catheter include improving self-care and adaptability, reducing the incidence of catheter-related complications, reducing the demand for medical consumables (such as drainage bags), reducing sexual life obstacles, reducing catheter-related lower urinary tract symptoms (frequency voiding, urgency, incontinence), and beneficial for patients to return to society [14, 15]. Therefore, for patients with bladder dysfunction, especially NB patients with increased PVR, CIC is the preferred treatment method. The common types of lower urinary tract dysfunction in NB patients and their definitions are shown in Table 4.1.

As can be seen from Table 4.1, not all NB patients are suitable for CIC, because the bladder dysfunction of patients varies, and with the development of the disease, the type of bladder dysfunction may also change. Therefore, it is necessary to regularly perform urodynamic evaluation of the patient's bladder function, record catheterization diary, and develop an appropriate catheterization plan. According to urodynamic performance, give full consideration.

The lower urinary tract symptoms of NB patients can manifest as urinary incontinence (UI) or bladder cannot completely empty and urinary retention caused by outlet obstruction, impaired detrusor contraction function, or poor bladder compliance.

For patients with detrusor hypoactivity/areflexia bladder, their urodynamic performance is as follows: the detrusor pressure during the filling phase may not change significantly, or it may show reduced bladder compliance; during the voiding phase, it shows reduced detrusor pressure or no significant contraction. Such patients can be divided into two situations: If the function of the urethral sphincter is normal or hyperactive,

Table 4.1 Common types of lower urinary tract dysfunction in NB patients

Diagnosis	Definition
Detrusor hypoactivity/areflexia bladder, also refers to inactive, low contractility bladder	The bladder cannot contract and empty due to damage to the nerves that control the bladder. The bladder fills with urine and continues to fill. When the bladder can no longer accommodate more urine, the urine will flow out through the urethra, resulting in overflow incontinence
Neurogenic detrusor overactivity (NDO, formerly known as detrusor reflex hyperactivity)	Overactivity of the bladder detrusor leads to uncontrollable, involuntary bladder contractions, commonly seen in nerve damage above the sacral spinal level
Detrusor areflexia	Due to nerve damage, the detrusor cannot contract, commonly seen in spinal shock or lesions above the brainstem. Patients of this type may experience urinary retention
Detrusor-sphincter dyssynergia (DSD)	Bladder outlet dysfunction, leading to loss of coordination between the bladder detrusor and the urethral sphincter. When the bladder contracts, the sphincter also contracts, affecting urine flow. The bladder cannot resist the closed sphincter and effectively empty, resulting in urinary retention. The bladder pressure of these patients is very high, causing urine to reflux to the ureter, eventually leading to kidney damage
Detrusor hyperactivity/hyperreflexia bladder with impaired bladder contraction function	Patients of this type are characterized by frequent ineffective involuntary detrusor contractions, unable to completely empty the bladder or only able to empty the bladder with effort (abdominal pressure, Crede maneuver, etc.)

the urethra is closed during voiding, and the bladder cannot generate effective pressure to counteract the resistance of the urethra; therefore it cannot effectively empty, resulting in a large amount of PVR. This may lead to overflow incontinence. This situation is the best indication for CIC. Another situation is when the patient's urethral sphincter function is impaired or combined with stress incontinence. These patients can use abdominal pressure or Crede maneuver to urinate. As long as the bladder pressure during voiding is within the normal range and can effectively empty the bladder, there is no need for auxiliary CIC treatment.

For patients with overactive detrusor, their urodynamic performance is as follows: involuntary contraction waves of the detrusor can be seen during the filling phase, or even terminal overactivity, leading to urge incontinence. It can also manifest as reduced bladder compliance; during the voiding phase, the contraction force of the detrusor may decrease, and the PVR in the bladder may increase. For such patients, oral drugs (M receptor blockers, β3 receptor agonists, etc.) should be the first choice to control overactive bladder (OAB) symptoms, to prevent bladder pressure from being too high, leading to VUR, and damaging upper urinary tract function [16–18]. If the OAB symptoms are controlled by drugs, and the patient also has reduced detrusor contraction force, increased PVR accompanied by VUR or abnormal voiding, such as incontinence, urinary retention, recurrent UTI, or increased PVR (adults >200 mL, children >50% of predicted maximum bladder capacity) with a tendency to various voiding abnormalities or UTI, it is necessary to perform partial CIC (catheterization once in the morning and once in the evening, i.e., after waking up and urinating in the morning and before going to bed at night, as detailed in the following text) and encourage more autonomous voiding.

For patients with areflexic detrusor, their symptoms and urodynamic results are similar to those of patients with low-activity bladder. If they cannot effectively empty the bladder, CIC treatment is also needed.

For DSD patients, the main urodynamic abnormality is abnormally high detrusor pressure during voiding, but no effective urine flow is formed. If bladder-urethral synchronous pressure measurement is performed, it can be found that the detrusor pressure and urethral pressure rise simultaneously. Therefore, the patient cannot effectively empty the bladder, and urinary retention occurs. For such patients, drugs (α receptor blockers) should be the first choice to relax the urethral sphincter. If the bladder cannot be effectively emptied after taking the drug, CIC treatment can be assisted [19].

4.1.2 Non-neurogenic Neurogenic Bladder

Non-neurogenic neurogenic bladder (NNB) is a voiding dysfunction caused by poor voiding habits and psychological or mental factors, without clear nerve damage factors. It is often accompanied by OAB, urinary retention, dysuria, and other clinical manifestations, also known as Hinman syndrome. The characteristic of these patients is that modern examination methods cannot find neurological defects or lesions, but the clinical symptoms and changes in bladder morphology are consistent with the changes of NB, and the results of UDS also suggest the existence of bladder-urethral dysfunction. For such patients, early detection and treatment are needed. Once the patient's bladder morphology has undergone significant changes, and even if the pathological factors are removed, it is difficult for the bladder function to fully recover to normal. For the treatment of NNB patients, eliminating the cause of the disease and correcting bad voiding habits, as well as psychological interventions, are important treatment methods. While treating the cause of the disease, the patient's urodynamic results and PVR can be judged. If there is a low-activity bladder and the bladder cannot effectively empty, CIC adjuvant treatment should be given. Those who still have the ability to urinate autonomously and have increased PVR should consider partial CIC [20–22].

Another situation is seen in bladder dysfunction caused by long-term lower urinary tract obstruction caused by prostate hyperplasia. Due to long-term obstruction, the bladder detrusor contraction function is impaired, the bladder morphology changes, and functionally it manifests as bladder emptying disorder, and therefore, its clinical manifestations are similar to NB. For such patients, the surgical result may not be ideal, or there are factors such as old age and multiple comorbidities that are not suitable for surgery; cystostomy and/or CIC treatment should be considered [7].

4.1.3 CIC After Bladder Urethral Surgery

CIC is often used as an auxiliary treatment method after various bladder urethral surgeries, with the aim of preventing urinary system infections and protecting upper urinary tract function and winning time for the recovery of voiding function or for patient voiding training. After bladder augmentation (bladder autologous enlargement surgery or intestinal bladder enlargement surgery), a considerable part of patients cannot completely empty, leaving a large amount of PVR; CIC is the best solution. Urinary retention often requires CIC intervention after urethral suspension surgery. A considerable part of orthotopic neobladder patients has found an increase in PVR during long-term follow-up. If it exceeds 200 mL, CIC auxiliary treatment is needed to assist bladder emptying, prevent urinary system infections, and protect upper urinary tract function.

1. After bladder augmentation: For severe OAB, radiation cystitis, NB combined with low compliance bladder, resulting in a severe reduction in functional bladder capacity, and even combined with reflux, bladder augmentation can be performed (autologous bladder enlargement, ureteral bladder enlargement, intestinal bladder enlargement, biological patch bladder enlargement). The purpose of bladder augmentation is to increase bladder capacity while reducing bladder pressure, protecting upper urinary tract function. However, after the surgery, due to the original factors (NB) or the enlargement material do not have contraction function, if abdominal pressure or Crede maneuver voiding cannot effectively empty the bladder, CIC treatment is needed.

2. Post-intestinal orthotopic neobladder: For patients who have undergone radical cystectomy + intestinal replacement/orthotopic neobladder due to bladder tumors or other reasons, the new bladder does not have contraction function. Patients need to urinate through abdominal pressure or Crede maneuver. If the bladder cannot effectively empty, and there is a large amount of PVR, CIC may be required.
3. Post-urethral suspension surgery: For patients with stress urinary incontinence who have undergone urethral suspension surgery (females) or artificial sphincter (males), if postoperative dysuria and increased PVR occur, and after dilation of the urethra, there is still a large amount of PVR, CIC treatment can be considered.
4. Post-lower urinary tract obstruction surgery: For patients who have undergone surgery due to benign prostatic hyperplasia, bladder neck contraction, or urethral stricture, if the urinary tract obstruction has been relieved, but the bladder cannot effectively empty due to impaired detrusor contraction function and there is a large amount of PVR, CIC treatment can be considered [23].
5. Prevention of urethral stricture after urethral surgery: Urethral stricture often occurs after urethral plastic surgery. Patients who need frequent urethral dilation can undergo CIC to prevent the occurrence of urethral stricture. There are many methods to prevent urethral stricture after urethral surgery, and CIC is one of the most commonly used methods. The incidence of urethral stricture with and without the use of CIC after urethral surgery is 9% and 31%.

4.1.4 CIC as an Adjunctive Treatment

For example, temporary urinary retention caused by improper use of M receptor blockers or botulinum toxin, if conservative or drug treatment is ineffective, and the patient cannot tolerate the indwelling catheter, CIC can be considered as an adjunctive treatment. For patients with high detrusor reflex and impaired bladder contraction function, their urodynamic performance is as follows: involuntary contraction waves of the detrusor can be seen during the filling phase, even terminal overactivity, leading to urge urinary incontinence, and it may also show reduced bladder compliance; but during the voiding phase, the detrusor contraction function is impaired, and the bladder cannot effectively empty, leading to an increase in PVR. Such patients should also choose drug treatment (M receptor blockers, β3 receptor agonists, etc.) as the first choice. After controlling OAB symptoms, if the PVR significantly increases, partial CIC should be considered (see later).

If the following situations exist, and it is not difficult to insert a catheter into bladder, the CIC can also be considered: (1) BOO; (2) benign prostatic hyperplasia; (3) urethral stricture; (4) prune belly syndrome; (5) bladder exstrophy; (6) trauma; (7) other diseases causing BOO [19].

4.2 Contraindications of CIC

There are few absolute contraindications for CIC, mainly persistent high pressure in the bladder, which requires continuous bladder drainage to avoid kidney damage. In the absence of professional nursing assistance, due to poor hand flexibility, it is not easy to complete CIC, which is a relative contraindication. Other contraindications mainly occur in the following situations [24, 25]:

1. Neurological or psychological factors: Patients with mental disorders or severe autonomic reflexes that prevent them from performing CIC or cooperating with CIC. For those with dementia, patients cannot perform catheterization themselves, and performing CIC loses the meaning of saving medical expenses and helping patients return to society.
2. Physical mobility factors: Patients with paralysis, upper limb mobility disorders, tremors, etc. are not suitable for self-CIC.

3. Infection factors: Complications such as pyuria and other severe urethritis, cystitis, urethral abscess, etc.
4. Local factors: The following are situations where the catheter cannot be inserted or the insertion of the catheter will worsen the condition or affect the treatment of the disease: (a) The patient has bladder neck constriction, urethral stenosis, deformity, etc., which makes it impossible to insert the catheter into the bladder or pass safely. (b) There is a fistula in the urethra. (c) Severe spasm of the pelvic floor muscles or urethral sphincter and dysfunction of the urethral sphincter may cause difficulty in inserting or removing the catheter. (d) Urethral injury, bleeding. (e) Bladder contraction or other reasons cause a significant reduction in effective bladder capacity, which is not suitable for CIC, and bladder enlargement surgery should be performed first before CIC. (f) Severe prostatic hyperplasia and the catheter cannot be inserted. (g) Severe autonomic nerve abnormal reflex still exists after treatment. (h) Abnormal penile erection [26].

In summary, as long as we strictly follow the indications, CIC is a good, minimally invasive, simple, and economical method for treating bladder voiding disorders. It is mainly used for various reasons that cause a large amount of PVR, but it may cause some complications. Therefore, in order to achieve the best results, a detailed imaging and urodynamic assessment should be conducted on the patient before determining the implementation of CIC to avoid unnecessary complications.

References

1. Engberg S, Clapper J, Mcnichol L, et al. Current evidence related to intermittent catheterization: a scoping review [J]. J Wound Ostomy Continence Nurs. 2020;47(2):140–65. https://doi.org/10.1097/won.0000000000000625.
2. Lamin E, Newman DK. Clean intermittent catheterization revisited [J]. Int Urol Nephrol. 2016;48(6):931–9. https://doi.org/10.1007/s11255-016-1236-9.
3. Szymanski KM, Fuchs M, Mcleod D, et al. Probability of bladder augmentation, diversion and clean intermittent catheterization in classic bladder exstrophy: a 36-year, multi-institutional, retrospective cohort study [J]. J Urol. 2019;202(6):1256–62. https://doi.org/10.1097/ju.0000000000000552.
4. Merhej S, Masri H, Moukarzel M, et al. [Augmentation cystoplasty and intermittent catheterization in neurogenic bladder] [J]. J Med Liban. 1994;42(3):109–11.
5. Myers JB, Lenherr SM, Stoffel JT, et al. The effects of augmentation cystoplasty and botulinum toxin injection on patient-reported bladder function and quality of life among individuals with spinal cord injury performing clean intermittent catheterization [J]. Neurourol Urodyn. 2019;38(1):285–94. https://doi.org/10.1002/nau.23849.
6. Bauer SB, Choung K, Sable P, et al. The impact of clean intermittent catheterization on students and families in the school environment [J]. Neurourol Urodyn. 2023;42(8):1702–11. https://doi.org/10.1002/nau.25271.
7. Lapides J, Diokno AC, Silber SJ, Lowe BS. Clean, intermittent self-catheterization in the treatment of urinary tract disease [J]. J Urol. 2017;197(2S):S122–4.
8. Katrancha ED. Clean intermittent catheterization in the school setting [J]. J Sch Nurs. 2008;24(4):197–204. https://doi.org/10.1177/1059840508319865.
9. Rondon A. When to start clean intermittent catheterization (CIC) in children with neurogenic bladder dysfunction [J]. Int Braz J Urol. 2022;48(1):52–3. https://doi.org/10.1590/s1677-5538.Ibju.2020.0989.1.
10. Corcos J. Evaluation and treatment of neurogenic bladder [M]. Beijing: People's Medical Publishing House; 2010.
11. Stein R, Bogaert G, Dogan HS, et al. EAU/ESPU guidelines on the management of neurogenic bladder in children and adolescent part I diagnostics and conservative treatment [J]. Neurourol Urodyn. 2020;39(1):45–57. https://doi.org/10.1002/nau.24211.
12. Li Y, Wen Y, He X, et al. Application of clean intermittent catheterization for neurogenic bladder in infants less than 1 year old [J]. NeuroRehabilitation. 2018;42(4):377–82. https://doi.org/10.3233/nre-172366.
13. Place J. Advances in clean intermittent self-catheterisation: impact on trauma and urinary tract infections [J]. Br J Nurs. 2023;32(Sup18):S5–7. https://doi.org/10.12968/bjon.2023.32.Sup18.S5.
14. Herbert AS, Welk B, Elliott CS. Internal and external barriers to bladder management in persons with neurologic disease performing intermittent catheterization [J]. Int J Environ Res Public Health. 2023;20(12):6079. https://doi.org/10.3390/ijerph20126079.
15. Joshi AD, Shukla A, Chawathe V, Gaur AK. Clean intermittent catheterization in long-term management of neurogenic bladder in spinal cord injury: patient perspective and experiences [J]. Int J

Urol. 2022;29(4):317–23. https://doi.org/10.1111/iju.14776.
16. Dmochowski R, Chapple C, Gruenenfelder J, et al. The effects of age, gender, and postvoid residual volume on catheterization rates after treatment with onabotulinumtoxinA for overactive bladder [J]. Eur Urol Open Sci. 2023;57:98–105. https://doi.org/10.1016/j.euros.2023.09.013.
17. Jiang M, Deng J, Zhou G, et al. Risk factors for recurrent urinary tract infection in children with neurogenic bladder following clean intermittent catheterization [J]. Urology. 2022;164:224–9. https://doi.org/10.1016/j.urology.2021.12.027.
18. Kennelly M, Green L, Alvandi N, et al. Clean intermittent catheterization rates after initial and subsequent treatments with onabotulinumtoxinA for non-neurogenic overactive bladder in real-world clinical settings [J]. Curr Med Res Opin. 2018;34(10):1771–6. https://doi.org/10.1080/03007995.2018.1443061.
19. Newman DK, Willson MM. Review of intermittent catheterization and current best practices [J]. Urol Nurs. 2011;31(1):12–28, 48; quiz 29.
20. Buchter ML, Kjellberg J, Ibsen R, et al. Burden of illness among intermittent catheter users with non-neurogenic urinary retention in Denmark [J]. Expert Rev Pharmacoecon Outcomes Res. 2023;23(4):409–18. https://doi.org/10.1080/14737167.2023.2181793.
21. Welk B, Lenherr S, Santiago-Lastra Y, et al. Differences in the incidence of urinary tract infections between neurogenic and non-neurogenic bladder dysfunction individuals performing intermittent catheterization [J]. Neurourol Urodyn. 2022;41(4):1002–11. https://doi.org/10.1002/nau.24914.
22. Barken KB, Vaabengaard R. A scoping review on the impact of hydrophilic versus non-hydrophilic intermittent catheters on UTI, QoL, satisfaction, preference, and other outcomes in neurogenic and non-neurogenic patients suffering from urinary retention [J]. BMC Urol. 2022;22(1):153. https://doi.org/10.1186/s12894-022-01102-8.
23. Kamei J, Fujimura T. Urinary tract infection in patients with lower urinary tract dysfunction [J]. J Infect Chemother. 2023;29(8):744–8. https://doi.org/10.1016/j.jiac.2023.04.019.
24. Sorokin I, De E. Options for independent bladder management in patients with spinal cord injury and hand function prohibiting intermittent catheterization [J]. Neurourol Urodyn. 2015;34(2):167–76. https://doi.org/10.1002/nau.22516.
25. De Castro R, Fouda Neel KA, Alshammari AM, et al. Clean intermittent catheterization in Saudi children. Suggestion for a common protocol [J]. Saudi Med J. 2000;21(11):1016–23.
26. Clinical Advisory Board for Intermittent Catheterization. Clean intermittent catheterization: guidelines for healthcare professionals [J/OL]. 2013.

5 CIC Is Not as Terrifying and Complicated as Imagined

Jian-Guo Wen

Those who are unfamiliar with CIC often think it is a terrifying, difficult, and painful procedure. In fact, CIC is very simple, and it will not feel terrifying and painful after getting used to it. Every day, thousands of adult and child patients around the world are doing CIC. Most patients or their families can master the catheterization method after a few minutes of simple training [1].

CIC does not require strictly sterile.

Cleaning refers to the cleaning of the urethral catheters used, cleaning the perineum and urethral orifice with clean water, and washing hands with soap or hand sanitizer before catheterization. It does not need to be performed by medical staff in the hospital, the catheter does not need to be left in the bladder, the catheterization items can be carried by the patient, and the catheter can be inserted into the bladder through the urethra at any time when needed, reducing the dependence on urine drainage auxiliary equipment and utensils [2].

The purpose of CIC is to simulate physiological states to regularly fill and empty the bladder, prevent overfilling, and help maintain bladder capacity and restore bladder contractile function; regularly expel PVR, reduce urinary and reproductive system infections, and reduce the risk of urinary tract stones; and make the bladder intermittent expansion, protect bladder and kidney function, and improve sexual function and fertility, as well as patient's independence and quality of life [3].

J.-G. Wen (✉)
Pediatric Urodynamic Center/Department of Urology, First Affiliated Hospital of Zhengzhou University, Zhengzhou, China

5.1 Sterile Catheterization

In order to gain a deeper understanding of CIC, it is necessary to understand sterile catheterization (SC). SC refers to the method of inserting a catheter into the bladder through the urethra to drain urine under strict sterile operation. Urethral catheterization can easily cause iatrogenic infections, such as damage to the bladder and urethral mucosa caused by improper operation during catheterization, contamination of catheterization materials used, and violation of aseptic principles during operation, all of which can lead to urinary system infections. Therefore, when catheterizing a patient, it is necessary to strictly adhere to the principles and procedures of sterile technique [4]. Aseptic catheterization should be performed by professional medical staff within medical institutions, using sterile techniques during catheterization, including wearing masks, hats, sterile gloves, using disinfectant solution for disinfection, and using sterile catheterization kits, sterile catheters, etc. [5].

J.-G. Wen (ed.), *Progress in Clean Intermittent Catheterization*, Experts' Perspectives on Medical Advances, https://doi.org/10.1007/978-981-97-5021-4_5

5.1.1 Purpose of Catheterization

(1) To drain urine for patients with urinary retention, to alleviate pain. (2) To assist in clinical diagnosis, such as obtaining uncontaminated urine samples for bacterial culture; measuring bladder capacity, pressure, and PVR; performing urethral or bladder radiography, etc. (3) To perform bladder chemotherapy for patients with bladder tumors.

5.1.2 Pre-procedure Preparation [6]

Assess the patient and explain: (1) Assessment: the patient's age, condition, clinical diagnosis, purpose of catheterization, state of consciousness, vital signs, coprocedure level, psychological state, self-care ability, bladder fullness, perineal skin and mucous membrane condition and cleanliness. (2) Explanation: Explain to the patient and their family about the purpose, method, precautions, and key points of procedure for catheterization. Depending on the patient's self-care ability, instruct them to clean the perineum.

Patient preparation: (1) The patient and their family understand the purpose, significance, process, precautions, and key points of coprocedure for catheterization. (2) Clean the perineum and prepare for catheterization. If the patient is unable to care for themselves, assist them in cleaning the perineum.

Nurse preparation: Neatly dressed, nails trimmed, hands washed, mask worn.

Equipment preparation: (1) Top layer of the treatment cart: Disposable catheterization kit (sterilized catheterization kit, including preliminary disinfection, secondary disinfection, and catheterization items. Preliminary disinfection items include a small tray, a bag containing several disinfectant cotton balls, tweezers, gauze, disposable gloves. Secondary disinfection and catheterization items include a curved tray, a bag containing four disinfectant cotton balls, two tweezers, a 10 mL syringe with sterile liquid, a bag of lubricant-soaked cotton balls, a specimen bottle, gauze, a urine collection bag, a square tray, a hole towel, sterile gloves, an outer package treatment towel). A suitable size sterile catheter, hand disinfectant, curved tray, disposable pad or small rubber sheet and treatment towel set, bath towel. (2) Bottom layer of the treatment cart: Bedpan and bedpan towel, household waste bin, medical waste bin. (3) Others: Prepare screens as appropriate according to the environment.

Environment preparation: Close doors, windows, curtains, or screens to shield the patient as appropriate. Maintain an appropriate room temperature. Sufficient lighting or adequate illumination.

5.1.3 Procedure Steps [7]

5.1.3.1 Check and Explain

Place the patient's belongings next to the bed, verify the patient's bed number and name, and explain the purpose of the procedure and related matters to the patient again. (Key points and explanations: Confirm the patient; obtain the patient's cooperation).

5.1.3.2 Preparation

Move the bedside chair to the same side of the bed, place the bedpan on the chair at the foot of the bed, and open the bedpan cover. (Key points and explanations: Facilitate operation; save time and effort.) Loosen the quilt at the foot of the bed, help the patient remove the pants on the opposite side, cover the near side of the leg, and cover with a bath towel. The opposite leg is covered with a quilt. (Key points and explanations: Prevent catching cold.)

5.1.3.3 Prepare the Position

Assist the patient to take a supine position with bent knees, slightly spread legs, and expose the vulva. (Key points and explanations: Facilitate nurse operation.)

5.1.3.4 Pad

Place a small rubber sheet and treatment pad under the patient's buttocks, place a curved tray near the vulva, disinfect both hands, open the catheterization package, take out the initial disinfection items, the operator puts on gloves on one hand, and pour the disinfectant cotton ball into the small square tray. (Key points and explanations: Protect the bed sheet from contamination; ensure the sterility of the procedure, and prevent the occurrence of infection.)

5.1.3.5 Disinfection and Catheterization

Disinfect and catheterize according to the anatomical characteristics of the male and female patient's urethra [8].

Female patient: (1) Initial disinfection: The operator holds the tweezers with one hand to disinfect the mons pubis and labia majora with the disinfectant cotton ball, and the other hand with gloves separates the labia majora and disinfects the labia minora and the urethral orifice; the dirty cotton ball is placed in the curved tray; after disinfection, remove the gloves, and place them in the curved tray; move the curved tray and the small square tray to the foot of the bed. (Key points and explanations: Each cotton ball is used only once; the tweezers should not touch the anal area; the order of disinfection is from outside to inside, from top to bottom.) (2) Open the catheterization package: After disinfecting both hands with hand sanitizer, place the catheterization package between the patient's legs, and open the treatment pad according to the principles of aseptic technique. (Key points and explanations: Instruct the patient not to move their limbs, maintain the placed position, and avoid contamination of the sterile area.) (3) Put on sterile gloves; spread the hole towel: Take out the sterile gloves, put on the sterile gloves according to the principles of aseptic technique, take out the hole towel, spread it on the patient's vulva, and expose the perineum. (Key points and explanations: The hole towel and the treatment towel form a continuous sterile area, expand the sterile area, facilitate aseptic procedure, and avoid contamination.) (4) Arrange the materials and lubricate the catheter: Arrange the materials in the order of procedure, take out the catheter, lubricate the front section of the catheter with a lubricant-soaked cotton ball, connect the catheter and the drainage tube of the urine collection bag as needed, and place the disinfected cotton ball in the curved tray. (Key points and explanations: This facilitates procedure; lubricating the catheter can reduce the irritation of the catheter to the mucous membrane and the resistance during catheter insertion.) (5) Disinfect again: Place the curved tray at the vulva, use one hand to separate and fix the labia minora, and use the other hand to hold the tweezers to clamp the disinfected cotton ball, and disinfect the urethral orifice, both sides of the labia minora and the urethral orifice. Place the dirty cotton balls, curved tray, and tweezers in the curved tray at the end of the bed. (Key points and explanations: The order of disinfection is from inside to outside, from top to bottom; each cotton ball is used only once to avoid re-contamination of the disinfected area; when disinfecting the urethral orifice, pause for a moment to fully utilize the disinfectant effect.); (6) Catheterization: Place the square tray next to the hole towel, instruct the patient to open their mouth and breathe, use the tweezers on the other side to hold the catheter, and gently insert it into the urethra, 4–6 cm; when you see urine flowing out, insert another 1 cm or so, release the hand fixing the labia minora, and move it down to fix the catheter, and guide the urine into the urine collection bag or square tray. (Key points and explanations: Breathing with the mouth open can relax the patient's muscles and the urethral sphincter, which helps with catheter insertion; the action of inserting the catheter should be gentle to avoid damaging the urethral mucosa.)

Male patient: (1) Preliminary disinfection: The operator holds the tweezers in one hand to clamp the disinfected cotton ball for preliminary disinfection, in the order of the pubic area, penis, and scrotum. The other hand wearing a glove takes a sterile gauze to wrap the penis and pushes the foreskin back to expose the urethral orifice, wiping the urethral orifice, glans, and coronal sulcus in a rotating motion from the urethral orifice outward and backward. Place the dirty cotton balls and gauze in the curved tray; after disinfection, move the small square tray and curved tray to the end of the bed and remove the gloves. (Key points and explanations: Each cotton ball is used only once; disinfect from the base of the penis to the urethral orifice; the foreskin and coronal sulcus can easily hide dirt, so careful wiping should be done to prevent infection.) (2) Open the catheter package: After disinfecting both hands with hand sanitizer, place the catheter package between the patient's legs, and open the treatment towel according to the principles of aseptic technique. (Key points and explanations: Instruct the patient not to move their limbs, maintain the position, and avoid contamination of the sterile area.) (3) Wear sterile gloves and spread the hole towel: Take out the sterile gloves, wear them according to the principles of aseptic technique, take out the hole towel, spread it on the patient's vulva, and expose the penis. (Key points and explanations: The hole towel and treatment towel form a continuous sterile area, expanding the sterile area, facilitating aseptic procedure, and avoiding contamination.) (4) Arrange the materials and lubricate the catheter: Arrange the materials in the order of procedure, take out the catheter, lubricate the front section of the catheter with a lubricant-soaked cotton ball, connect the catheter and the drainage tube of the urine collection bag as needed, place it in the square tray, and place the disinfected cotton ball in the curved tray. (Key points and explanations: This facilitates procedure; avoid contaminating the environment with urine.) (5) Disinfection again: Move the curved tray to the vulva, use one hand to wrap the penis with gauze, and push the foreskin back, exposing the urethral orifice. The other hand holds the tweezers to clamp the disinfectant cotton ball for disinfection of the urethra opening, glans, and coronal sulcus again. Dirty cotton balls and tweezers are placed in the curved tray at the end of the bed. (Key points and explanations: This disinfection sequence is from the inside out; each cotton ball is used only once to avoid re-contamination of the disinfected area.) (6) Catheterization: One hand continues to use sterile gauze to fix the penis and lift it, making it a 60° angle with the abdominal wall, place the square tray next to the hole towel, instruct the patient to open their mouth and breathe, use the other tweezers to hold the catheter, and gently insert it into the urethra 20–22 cm, until urine flows out. Then insert another 1–2 cm, and guide the urine into the urine collection bag or the square tray. (Key points and explanations: The urethra of adult males is 17–20 cm long, with two bends: the prepubic bend and the infrapubic bend. There are three narrow parts: the external orifice of the urethra, the membranous part, and the internal orifice. Making the prepubic bend disappear is beneficial for catheter insertion; the action of inserting the catheter should be gentle, and when it reaches the narrow part of the urethra, avoid using excessive force or speed to damage the urethral mucosa.)

5.1.3.6 Clamp the Tube and Pour Out the Urine

When the urine fills 2/3 of the square tray, clamp the end of the catheter, pour the urine into the bedpan, then open the catheter to continue urination, or drain the urine into the urine collection bag to the appropriate amount [9]. If necessary, retain a urine sample. (Key points and explanations: Pay attention to the patient's reaction, and ask about their feelings.)

5.1.3.7 Post-procedure Handling

(1) After catheterization, gently pull out the catheter, remove the hole towel, clean the vulva, dispose of the catheterization items in the medical waste bin, remove the small rubber sheet and treatment towel under the patient's buttocks, and place them on the lower layer of the treatment cart. Remove gloves, disinfect hands with hand sanitizer, and assist the patient in putting on their pants. (Key points and explanations: Make the patient comfortable; protect the patient's privacy.) (2) Clean up the items, measure the urine volume, label the urine sample, and send it for inspection. (3) Disinfect both hands, and record. (Key points and explanations: Record the time of catheterization, the amount of urine drained, and the patient's condition and reaction [10].)

5.1.4 Precautions for Sterile Catheterization [11]

1. Strictly implement the checking system and principles of sterile procedure.
2. During the procedure, pay attention to protecting the patient's privacy, and take appro-

priate warming measures to prevent the patient from catching a cold.

3. For patients with highly distended and extremely weak bladders, the first urination should not exceed 1000 mL. Excessive urination can cause a sharp drop in intra-abdominal pressure, a large amount of blood stagnation in the abdominal cavity, leading to a drop in blood pressure and collapse; in addition, a sudden drop in bladder pressure can also cause the bladder mucosa to become severely congested, resulting in hematuria.
4. In elderly women, the urethral orifice retracts, so careful observation and identification should be made when catheterizing to avoid mistakenly entering the vagina.
5. When catheterizing female patients, if the catheter mistakenly enters the vagina, a sterile catheter should be replaced and then re-catheterized.
6. To avoid damage and infection of the urinary system, it is necessary to understand the anatomical characteristics of the male and female urethra.

5.2 CIC Notice [12]

CIC requires the patient to have sufficient bladder capacity and normal urinary bladder control. In addition, it requires the patient and family members (caregivers) to have strong learning and hands-on abilities and a deep understanding of the disease and to actively cooperate with treatment, with good compliance.

CIC has certain limitations and risks. Firstly, this technique is not a routine procedure in undergraduate nursing textbooks, there is no specific tutorial, and this lacks evidence-based medical evidence and is not accepted by most medical staff in actual clinical promotion work, let alone recognized and understood by many patients and their families, which can easily lead to medical disputes. Secondly, CIC often accompanies the patient for life, some patients must completely rely on the assistance of caregivers to complete, and there are certain restrictions on the specific time of catheterization, increasing the economic and care burden of individuals and families, requiring patients and caregivers to have good compliance. Furthermore, catheterization requires certain professional knowledge and operational skills, and implementing CIC requires professional training from medical staff and continuous self-learning to master the correct procedure methods. Finally, catheterization is an invasive and traumatic procedure, which may cause pain, cause urethral injury, bleeding, and complications such as the formation of false passages, urethral stricture, fever, infection, etc., and also requires equipped facilities, barrier-free bathrooms, or appropriate areas. However, compared with long-term indwelling catheters and bladder fistulas, CIC is safer, more reliable, and convenient.

5.3 CIC Implementation Steps

5.3.1 Patient Assessment and Training

5.3.1.1 Assessment

Patient's age, condition, clinical diagnosis, purpose of catheterization, consciousness status, vital signs, self-care ability, hand mobility, vision, cooperation level, psychological status, compliance, bladder and urethral function, and perineal skin and mucosal conditions, etc., to determine whether the patient is suitable for CIC and decide whether the catheterization is performed by the patient or the caregiver.

5.3.1.2 Explanation

Explain the purpose and significance of CIC to patients and caregivers based on the different executing entities of CIC, using models to explain the anatomical structure and function of the urinary system, catheterization procedure and procedures, precautions, cooperation points, complications and treatment principles, follow-up reviews, etc. [13].

5.3.1.3 Training and Learning Methods

(1) Medical staff provide one-on-one live demonstrations and oral explanations to patients and their

families. (2) Patients or family members shall operate in person, and medical staff shall provide on-site guidance. (3) Organize to watch professional website catheterization videos. (4) Join the CIC-related official account, patient club, and WeChat discussion group. (5) Distribute promotional materials, establish specialized nursing clinics for consultation, and create a learning and communication platform for patients.

5.3.2 CIC Procedure

5.3.2.1 Preparation and Operation

1. Environment preparation: Choose a clean, spacious, bright, safe, unobstructed, quiet, private, warm environment. The home bathroom should be equipped with dedicated storage cabinets, hooks, etc.
2. Material preparation: Suitable size of sterile or clean catheter, transparent urine collection container or urine bag with scale, water-soluble lubricant, gauze or tissue, disposable wet wipes, hand mirror (for women, better with magnification), movable light source, disposable pad, soap or antibacterial hand wash, no-wash quick hand sanitizer, sterile gloves, when necessary, compound lidocaine cream (for patients sensitive to pain), waste bin, etc. The placement should be convenient for the patient and in the order of procedure.
3. Hand washing: Hands are the main medium for CIC to cause urinary system infections, and strict hand washing is an important means to prevent cross-infection. The operator should trim their nails regularly, and wash their hands before and after catheterization with soap or hand wash, rinse with clean water, and dry with clean gauze or tissue. When there is no condition for hand washing, you can use no-wash quick hand sanitizer or wet wipes to wipe your hands. It is recommended to use the seven-step hand washing method (Fig. 5.1).
4. Remove clothing: Adopt the most comfortable and convenient position for catheterization, clothes and pants should be loose and easy to put on and take off, and for patients with mobility difficulties, paraplegics, it is best to have an opening in the crotch of the pants.
5. Cleaning the perineum and urethral orifice: The female urethra is short, and the various orifices of the perineum are close to each other, making cross-infection easy. Therefore, for females, during menstruation, urinary and reproductive system infections, incontinence, excessive perineal secretions,

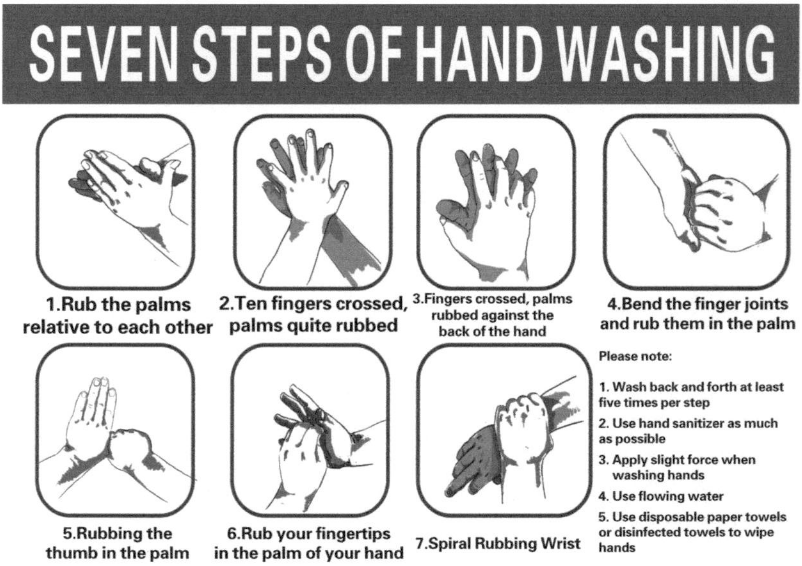

Fig. 5.1 Seven steps of hand washing

incontinent dermatitis, perineal trauma, post-operative, and radiation damage patients, warm water should be used multiple times to wipe or rinse the perineum before CIC. When wiping, start from the least contaminated area, change the wet wipe after each wipe, and do not reuse the wet wipe. The order of wiping is the labia, urethral and vagina orifice, and anus, so that the skin and mucous membranes around the perineum and urethral orifice are clean and dry, to prevent bacteria from spreading to the urethral orifice. The order of cleaning for male patients is the pubic mound, penis, and scrotum. When cleaning the penis, the foreskin should be completely turned back to expose the urethral orifice, and the urethral orifice, glans, and coronal sulcus should be wiped in a rotating motion from the urethral orifice outward and backward. The movements during the cleaning process should be gentle, reduce exposure, pay attention to warmth, and protect the patient's privacy [14].

6. Lubrication and use of the catheter: Depending on the different environments of home, working places, and school toilets, hang the catheter packaging bag on the hook of the bathroom door or wall for easy access by the patient. If a hydrophilic coating catheter that needs to be hydrated is used, open the packaging, and pour in warm boiled water or sterile saline (follow the instructions), and wait for the recommended duration. If a pre-lubricated hydrophilic catheter is used, hang the packaging bag directly next to the patient for use. If a non-coated catheter is used, a water-soluble lubricant can be selectively used, applied to the surface of the catheter or the urethral orifice.
7. Placement of the catheter: According to the different anatomical structures of the male and female urethra, gently insert the catheter into the bladder through the urethra. When urine flows out, it proves that the catheter has entered the bladder.
8. Drainage of urine: Completely drain the urine into the toilet or urine collection container.
9. Removal of the catheter: Slowly pull out the catheter. Before the catheter is completely pulled out, fold the end of the catheter to prevent urine from dripping out and causing contamination.
10. Place the urine collector on a flat surface; observe the characteristics of the urine; check for hematuria, pyuria, whether there is white flocculent turbidity, whether there is a foul smell, etc.; and record it in the voiding diary.

5.3.2.2 Catheterization Frequency [15]

The number of CIC catheterizations is determined by the amount of urine. Adults should control the amount of urine drainage volume not to exceed 400 mL per catheterization when the bladder is emptied. In addition, the number of catheterizations varies greatly among patients and is related to the amount of water the patient drinks. Usually, patients need to catheterize four to six times a day. The amount of catheterization for infants and children can be estimated using the formula for the maximum normal bladder volume [age (years) × 30 mL + 30 mL] [16].

5.3.3 General Precautions and Handling of Special Situations in CIC

5.3.3.1 General Precautions

1. Regularly perform CIC based on PVR, and avoid waiting until the patient feels an urgent need to urinate or experiences incontinence.
2. If you encounter obstacles during catheterization, pause for 5–10 seconds, take a deep breath, and withdraw the catheter by 3 cm, and then slowly reinsert it.
3. If you encounter resistance when removing the catheter, it may be due to urethral spasms. Wait for 5–10 minutes before removing the catheter.
4. Vaginal packing can affect the insertion of the catheter. Therefore, women should remove any vaginal packing before catheterization. If the catheter is accidentally inserted

into the vagina, a new catheter should be used.

5. Be gentle when inserting the catheter, especially for male patients. Pay attention when the catheter passes through the narrow part of the urethral orifice, the curved part of the pubic symphysis, and the internal opening of the urethra, the patient is advised to take slow and deep breaths, and slowly insert the catheter. Avoid causing damage to the urethral mucosa by inserting too quickly or forcefully.
6. To reduce the risk of infection, a no-touch catheterization method can be advocated. Unlike traditional intermittent catheterization, after washing hands again, directly pick up the catheter packaging bag, pour out the sterilizing water in the bag, tear open the end of the catheter packaging bag exposing 10 cm of the catheter, and hold the packaging bag to insert the catheter into the urethral orifice. For female patients, insert the catheter 4–6 cm until urine flows out; for male patients, tear open the outer packaging bag three times, each time about 10 cm. During the entire process of catheter insertion, only touch the catheter packaging bag, not the catheter itself. You can also use the catheter's own protective sheath to avoid touching the catheter.
7. After successful catheterization, maintain the position of the catheter until all urine is drained. Do not immediately remove the catheter, but empty the bladder completely, leaving no PVR.
8. Regularly select appropriate catheterization frequency and timing based on PVR and water intake. The frequency of catheterization is affected by individual differences, generally four to six times a day. For patients who cannot urinate on their own due to complete urinary retention, catheterization should be performed five to six times a day. In adults, for patients who can urinate more than 100 mL between two catheterizations and have a bladder PVR of less than 300 mL, catheterization can be performed every 6 hours; for patients who can urinate more than 200 mL between two catheterizations and have a bladder PVR of less than 200 mL, catheterization can be performed every 8 hours; for patients with a bladder PVR of less than 80 mL or a bladder capacity of less than 20 mL, catheterization can be temporarily stopped.
9. It is recommended to use a portable bladder capacity meter to measure bladder capacity, achieving precise catheterization as needed. Especially for patients with overactive bladder, overflow incontinence, and low-pressure VUR, through non-invasive ultrasound technology, the bladder filling state and bladder capacity can be accurately measured, allowing patients to perform CIC before the urine volume over the safe bladder capacity.
10. It is recommended to follow the doctor's advice for regular follow-up by video urodynamic study during CIC. This allows patients to empty the bladder before incontinence occurs, before reaching a relatively safe bladder capacity, and before causing bladder vesicoureteral reflux, reducing the number of ineffective catheterizations, avoiding the occurrence of urinary tract infections, achieving the purpose of low-pressure urine storage, preventing bladder high pressure, vesicoureteral reflux damage to the kidneys, and also reducing patient suffering and caregiver catheterization burden.

During CIC in adults, water intake should be limited to between 1500 and 2000 mL and evenly distributed between 6 am and 8 pm, not exceeding 400 mL each time, and try to avoid drinking water 3 hours before bedtime. Try to avoid drinking diuretic beverages such as tea, coffee, and alcohol, and also try to avoid eating irritating, spicy foods, etc. After eating or drinking, please record the amount immediately and accurately. The daily intake and output must be balanced. If the target is not reached, appropriate adjustments should be made according to the situation [17].

The voiding diary is widely used in the research of various voiding dysfunctions. It is the simplest and non-invasive method to evaluate the lower urinary tract function. It is the basis for the choice of treatment strategies for NB. Families with conditions should actively record. The voiding diary can reflect many important information, such as the amount of each voiding, the interval of voiding, the total number of voidings and the total urine volume per day, bladder sensation, the number of incontinences, etc. (Table 5.1). Enter these data into the computer, analyze it with software, and calculate the average urine volume, frequency, average urine volume per minute, interval between two voidings, and urine volume at each specific period, and output a 24-hour time urine volume chart, total volume discharged throughout the day, the ratio of daytime and nighttime urine volume, etc. It is recommended to record the voiding diary for 7 days.

Routine UDS or VUDC: record PVR, maximum bladder pressure capacity, detrusor leakage point pressure, bladder compliance, relative bladder safety capacity, presence or absence of VUR, grading of VUR, bladder capacity and detrusor pressure at reflux, etc.

5.3.3.2 Handling of Special Situations in CIC

In the following situations, the doctor should be reported promptly for treatment: hematuria; failure to insert or remove the catheter; increased pain during catheter insertion that is unbearable; urinary irritation symptoms, dysuria, turbid urine, sediment, odor; lower abdominal pain, urethral burning sensation, etc.

How to handle these special situations in the CIC tutorial from The Clinical Advisory Board for Intermittent Catheterization (CABIC) is shown in Table 5.2.

5.3.3.3 Special Considerations for Different Genders and Infants in CIC

Female patients need to note that the female urethral orifice is located below the clitoris and above the vaginal opening and is thick and short (Fig. 5.2). Due to limited visibility, women often have difficulty identifying the location of the urethral orifice when self-catheterizing and may

Table 5.1 24-hour voiding/catheterization diary record table

Time date	Fluid intake	Leak volume	Self-voiding volume	Catheterization volume	Other
07:00					
08:00					
09:00					
10:00					
11:00					
12:00					
13:00					
14:00					
15:00					
16:00					
17:00					
18:00					
19:00					
20:00					
21:00					
22:00					
23:00					
24:00					

Note: (1) Fluid intake includes the water content of food and intravenous fluid volume; the total daily amount should not exceed 2000 mL at time of CIC, calculated according to the common food water content table. (2) Do not drink water 3 hours before sleep. (3) Please fill in the volume in the "self-voiding" column for autonomous voiding. (4) "Leakage" refers to wetting pants, bed sheets, and diapers, respectively, marked as "+," "++," "+++." (5) "Other" includes blood in urine (▼), smelly urine (※), turbidity (●), sediment (◆), difficulty in catheter insertion (⊙), fever (x), etc.; please fill in the symptoms symbols

Table 5.2 Methods for handling special situations in CIC

	Special situation	Treatment method
Difficulty in insertion/ catheter movement	Patient is too nervous	Distract the patient's attention and teach him to relax when the patient coughs or takes a deep breath, gently pressurize the insertion, urinary catheter with a syringe coated with lidocaine gel paste, wait for 3–5 minutes, and try again
	Catheter diameter is too big	Try a smaller catheter
	Catheter adheres to the surface of the urethra	Try other types/brands of catheters Try using a hydrophilic catheter instead of a traditional lubricating gel catheter to use more lubricant
No urine flow	Incomplete entry of catheter	The catheter should be further inserted into the bladder
	Positioning	Repositioning: Adjust the angle of the penis/ place a pillow under the female bone
	Sediment, mucus, clotted blood, tones	The bladder needs to be flushed or debris suctioned
	False passage	Remove and try again; seek medical attention promptly
	Catheter inserted into the vagina	Leave the catheter in place (to prevent the patient from inserting it incorrectly again), while inserting a new clean catheter into the urethra

mistakenly insert the catheter into the vagina. This can be avoided by using light and a mirror. The length of an adult female's urethra is usually 3–5 cm. Gently insert the catheter 4–6 cm during catheterization, and after seeing urine flow, insert another 1–2 cm.

Male patients need to note that the adult male urethra is 17–20 cm long, with two bends: the prepubic bend and the infrapubic bend; there are three narrow parts: the external orifice, the membranous part, and the internal orifice. When catheterizing, these anatomical features should be understood. When inserting the catheter, the penis should be lifted to form a 60° angle with the abdominal wall to eliminate the prepubic bend, allowing the catheter to be inserted smoothly, to a depth of about 20 cm, until urine flows out, and then proceed 1–2 cm further [18].

Infants and young children need to note that the anatomical feature of the urinary system in infants and young children is that the bladder is positioned higher. The newborn bladder is often pear-shaped and located above the pubic symphysis. The infant's bladder is close to the anterior abdominal wall and gradually descends into the pelvic cavity with age. The girl's urethra is short, with the newborn female infant's urethra length being 1.2–2.3 cm. The urethral length varies greatly at different ages in boys. The urethral length does not vary much in boys aged 1–6 years, being 6.2–6.4 cm, about 10.5 cm at 10 years old, and about 12.2 cm at 14 years old. It is recommended that beginners of CIC choose catheters with scale markings. Currently, there is a lack of precise data and research reports on the catheter insertion depth for infants and young children of all age groups both domestically and internationally. It is recommended that when catheterizing boys, the catheter should be slowly inserted until its tip surpasses the internal urethral orifice. Just as urine begins to flow out, continue to insert 2–3 cm further. At this time, the side hole of the catheter is above the internal urethral orifice in the bladder, allowing for smooth drainage of urine. When catheterizing female infants and young children, the catheter should first be inserted about 1.5 cm into the child's urethra. Once urine begins to flow out, insert another 0.5 cm. Or, the insertion depth can be determined according to the physiological length of the infant's urethra. The side hole of the catheter should be just at the bottom of the bladder, allowing for full drainage of PVR at the bottom of the bladder.

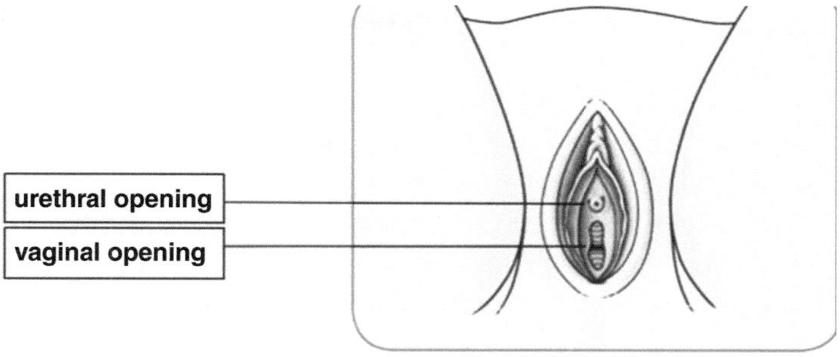

Fig. 5.2 The female urethral orifice is located below the clitoris and above the vaginal opening

5.3.4 Precautions for Catheterization in Patients with Prostate Hyperplasia

In patients with benign prostatic hyperplasia (BPH), the prostatic part of the urethra is elongated, and it is squeezed, deformed, twisted, and narrowed by the enlarged gland, resulting in increased urethral resistance. Common causes of catheterization failure in BPH include unskilled catheterization techniques, unclear understanding of the anatomical structure of the urethra under pathological conditions, insufficient use of lubricants, inappropriate types and models of catheters, high patient anxiety, discomfort and pain caused by the catheterization process itself, and lack of patient cooperation. These factors can cause the patient's overall muscle tension to increase, breathing to accelerate, and reflexive spasms and contractions of the pelvic floor muscles and urethral sphincter. Repeated forceful insertion and removal of the catheter can easily cause urethral mucosal edema, congestion, and urethral injury and even the formation of false passages, exacerbating urinary irritation symptoms after catheterization, making future catheterization more difficult, and even leading to the termination of the catheterization plan. To improve the success rate of catheterization in elderly men with BPH, in addition to choosing the right catheter, the technique of catheter insertion is also very important. The techniques and methods are introduced as follows.

5.3.4.1 Psychological Counseling

During the catheterization process, you can talk to the patient while operating to relieve tension and fear; effectively divert their attention. When the catheter encounters resistance in the posterior urethra, pause for a moment, and pull the catheter out a little; instruct the patient to take deep breaths while observing their expression, to reduce abdominal pressure; relax the external urethral sphincter, thereby reducing the resistance to catheter insertion; and opportunistically place the catheter smoothly into the bladder. The catheterization movement should be gentle and quick to reduce pain.

5.3.4.2 Prostate Curved Catheter (Curved Catheter)

For BPH patients, the curved catheter is the preferred choice. The head of this catheter is designed to be arc-shaped, thin, and sharp, which is beneficial for passing through the narrow parts of the urethral membrane and prostate in patients with prostate hyperplasia, and has more advantages than ordinary catheters. When someone else performs the CIC procedure, the patient takes the lithotomy position, the catheter is fully lubricated with sterile paraffin oil balls, and the penis is wrapped with gauze. The operator lifts the penis with his left hand to make it form a 60° angle with the abdominal wall, eliminating the pubic curvature. Hold the catheter with the right hand, insert the tip of the prostate catheter upward into the urethral opening, and when the catheter is nearly halfway inserted and feels blocked, it prompts the catheter to enter the second curved pubic curvature. At this time, put the penis down to make it about 90° with the abdomen, and continue to insert it into the bladder after the resistance disappears. The assistant can also gently massage the perineum, or lubricate the index finger and insert it into the patient's rectum, gently shake it up and down to relax the sphincter, and gently press the prostate upward and forward. The operator also appropriately adjusts the angle of insertion of the catheter so that the catheter can be smoothly pushed forward into the bladder along the fingertips.

5.3.4.3 Change the Type of Catheter

Choose a super smooth catheter. The friction coefficient of the super smooth catheter is much lower than that of the non-hydrophilic-coated catheter or ordinary catheter. It has excellent lubricity and biocompatibility, is easy to use, and comfortable to experience. It is recommended that beginners choose a catheter with a hydrophilic coating to reduce the risk of urethral injury and increase the success rate of catheter insertion.

5.3.4.4 Choose an Appropriate Size Catheter

If you encounter difficulties in catheterization, you can try again with a thinner catheter after the spasm is relieved.

5.3.4.5 Use Lubricant as Appropriate

In 2011, the Rehabilitation Nursing Professional Committee of the Chinese Rehabilitation Medical Association issued the "Neurogenic Bladder Care Guidelines," which clearly stated: When performing CIC with a non-coated or ordinary catheter, a lubricant must be used. Clinically, two types of lubricants are commonly used: sterile paraffin oil and water-soluble lubricants. Water-soluble lubricants are preferred. Using a lubricant to fully lubricate the entire catheter can reduce the irritation and friction of the catheter on the urethral mucosa and protect the urethral mucosa.

5.3.4.6 For Those Who Are Highly Sensitive to Pain, Use Sedatives and Analgesics as Appropriate

Lidocaine gel or ointment can be used as a lubricating analgesic. In addition to applying it to the tube body and the urethral orifice, try to make the lubricating analgesic enter the urethra to reach the urethral membrane, and keep it for 1–2 minutes before catheterization; a syringe without a needle can also be used to inject the gel into the urethra through the urethral orifice [19]. When the catheter enters the membranous urethra and encounters increased resistance, the assistant can inject the sedative analgesic through the end of the catheter while inserting the catheter, allowing the catheter to smoothly enter the bladder. Before catheterization, 2% lidocaine injection solution 5–10 mL can be injected into the urethra through the urethral orifice, then pinch the urethral orifice for surface infiltration anesthesia, and relax the external urethral sphincter; when the catheter is inserted into the membranous urethra, sterile paraffin oil 5–10 mL can be injected into the urethra to lubricate the urethra and reduce the resistance of catheterization. Gently insert the catheter with the right hand to prevent the catheter from bouncing back repeatedly. Insert about 1–2 cm each time, as it is easy to bend and break the catheter if it is too long. If repeated catheterization fails, seek medical attention in time.

5.3.5 Health Education [20]

Health education is a highly technical job, with a wide range of content and various forms. The targets of education include doctors, nurses, patients, and their families. Choose different health education content and methods according to the level of education, and provide personalized guidance.

5.3.5.1 Purpose

(1) To enable patients to master CIC technology, learn self-management, and reduce or eliminate fear and worry about CIC; (2) understand the significance of CIC in protecting the upper urinary tract and master the skills to adjust the timing of catheterization; (3) understand the level of recovery of voiding function and master the operation skills to avoid urinary tract infection; (4) understand the patient's understanding and mastery of CIC, train the patient and their family, provide targeted health guidance, increase the understanding of the disease, and enhance the confidence in treating the disease; (5) reduce catheterization complications.

5.3.5.2 Educational Objectives

For specialist doctor education: Doctors who guide CIC can come from urology, rehabilitation, obstetrics and gynecology, neurology, pediatrics, etc. Not all patients with NB are suitable for CIC, it is necessary to accurately grasp the indications and contraindications of CIC, and choose suitable patients; pay attention to the education of patients' related disease knowledge, so that they fully understand the necessity of CIC and the pros and cons of disease development; they need to have rich urodynamic professional knowledge, clarify the indications for UDS, guide patients to regularly follow up with video urodynamic study (VUDS), and based on the results of UDS, routine blood and urine tests, kidney function and urinary system ultrasound, etc., formulate personalized catheterization and treatment plans.

For specialist nurse education: Specialist nurses must undergo formal training and have rich relevant professional knowledge and mature experience in guiding CIC. They should instill in patients the concept of rehabilitation nursing that changes from "substitute care" to "self-care"; eliminate fear and resistance; provide patients with suitable teaching tools and standard CIC techniques; use media equipment to play CIC procedure videos and explain the purpose, key points, difficulties, precautions and observation, and handling of complications; use physical anatomical models or directly demonstrate one-on-one procedures for patients; and then let patients or family members demonstrate procedures, and nursing staff evaluate and correct their procedures to strengthen patients or family members' mastery of CIC procedures; help patients and family members establish the concept of clean procedure and master no-contact techniques, reducing the risk of CIC infection; for patients with poor acceptance and low cultural level, distribute CIC color page flowcharts; guide patients and family members to correctly record voiding (catheterization) diaries, keep patient records, guide the development of reasonable drinking plans, and accordingly provide timely and on-demand intermittent catheterization time and can assist doctors in improving the compliance of patients and parents of infants and young children.

For patient education: Patients should correctly view their own diseases; fully understand the advantages of CIC and possible complications; accept and recognize the necessity, long-term nature, and importance of CIC treatment with an optimistic attitude; and actively participate in the entire diagnosis and treatment process; they should be familiar with the anatomy of the urinary system and their own physiological structure, establish a clean concept, and master the CIC technique; strictly implement the drinking plan, strengthen self-bladder management, and reasonably adjust the frequency of catheterization; learn to observe the color, smell, characteristics, and volume of urine, etc.; if they find urine odor, turbid urine, flocculent matter, gross hematuria, pyuria, fever, general weakness and other symptoms of infection, they should follow up in time. Understand the clinical significance of UDS and routine blood and urine test parameters, such as PVR, maximum bladder pressure capacity, compliance, detrusor leak point pressure, safe bladder capacity, VUR, white blood cell count, kidney function, etc. Regularly re-examine UDS on time, communicate with the doctor in time, and change the treatment plan accordingly.

Education for patient's family or caregivers: the role of the patient's family or caregivers in the diagnosis and treatment process is indispensable. For special populations, such as infants, preschool children, the elderly, and patients with mobility difficulties, family members or caregivers are the executors of CIC. They not only need to learn necessary professional knowledge and master CIC techniques but also adjust according to the patient's specific situation. The attitude of family members and caregivers will have a great impact on the patient's psychology. They should enhance the patient's confidence to overcome the disease through language and actions, and let the patient believe that CIC is feasible, safe, and definitely effective. They must not show annoyance and should not cause long-term urinary retention due to negligence or irresponsibility, excessive PVR after long-term catheterization, urinary system infection, urethral injury, and other complications.

5.3.5.3 Health Education Methods and Forms

Strengthen knowledge education: standardize hand washing; pay attention to the convenience of the operation space and disinfection principles; strictly implement the clean operation principles during the procedure; before discharge, according to the patient's home situation, require family members to remodel the home environment, such as changing the furniture placement; prepare a spacious, bright, and easy-to-use equipment operation site; maintain indoor ventilation, and avoid catching a cold; maintain good personal hygiene habits; persist in rehabilitation exercises, enhance the body's resistance, and avoid infection.

Receive CIC nursing training before discharge, mainly one-on-one on-site guidance, face-to-face oral explanation, expert lectures, distribution of health manuals, and establishment of online communication platforms such as WeChat communication groups, WeChat public accounts, Twitter, QQ communication groups, telephone follow-ups, etc., to improve the patient's awareness of relevant knowledge and the degree of execution of medical orders; avoid running around, registering for medical treatment; reduce the patient's economic pressure and psychological burden; and establish a one-stop nursing model.

Regular follow-up: During CIC, if there is fever, VUR, febrile urinary system infection (body temperature $\geq$ 38 °C), difficulty in catheterization, urethral injury, severe gross hematuria, etc., you need to see a doctor at any time. Regular follow-ups can correct wrong procedures in time, solve encountered difficulties, and dynamically observe the disease. Improve and implement the follow-up system, adopt outpatient follow-up, telephone follow-up, and home visit follow-up methods, telephone follow-up 1 week after the patient is discharged, once a month thereafter, for 3 consecutive months. Talk to the patient or let the patient demonstrate the procedure, find out the existing problems and adjust the protocol and plan in time, encourage the patient to persist in the correct operation and training of bladder function, and enhance self-management ability. Regular VUDS is needed.

5.4 Technique for Adult Female CIC [21]

CIC can improve urinary incontinence symptoms in female patients, improve bladder function, facilitate normal sexual life, reduce urinary tract infections, achieve healthy kidney function, and improve quality of life. It is an effective measure for patients to manage their own bladder and gain greater independence in life and is the most effective control of their own bladder function. Adult female patients have specific characteristics and precautions when performing CIC due to their unique bladder urethral anatomical characteristics and psychological conditions.

5.4.1 Position Selection for Adult Female CIC

Adult female CIC requires the selection of an appropriate position. The correct position facilitates the smooth operation. The anatomical characteristics of the female urethra make it impossible for the patient to directly see the external urethral orifice. Choosing the appropriate position is conducive to successfully exposing the external urethral orifice and inserting the catheter. Therefore, patients should choose the appropriate position for CIC based on their condition, personal habits, environment, and bathroom facility conditions.

Position 1: Sitting in a wheelchair, placing both feet on the toilet ring or lifting one foot onto the toilet ring. The trick here is to place the catheter between the toilet seat and the base to secure the catheter, and then drain the urine into the toilet (Fig. 5.3a); or sit in a wheelchair with legs spread as far apart as possible (Fig. 5.3b). In this case, it is recommended to use a urine drainage bag or an intermittent catheterization kit, such as the LoFric Hydro-Kit. The above positions are suitable for patients with mobility impairments who rely on wheelchairs for daily life.

Position 2: Sitting on the toilet, legs spread apart, exposing the perineum (Fig. 5.3c).

Position 3: Sit on the bed with legs apart, bend one knee, and curl up one leg, fully exposing the genital area.

Position 4: Semi-sitting position, leaning against a pillow or quilt, raising the buttocks, bending the knees, feet facing each other, exposing the urethral orifice.

Position 5: Squatting on the squat toilet, legs apart, exposing the perineum.

Position 6: Standing position, one leg raised and propped on the edge of the toilet or stool, exposing the urethral orifice (Fig. 5.3d).

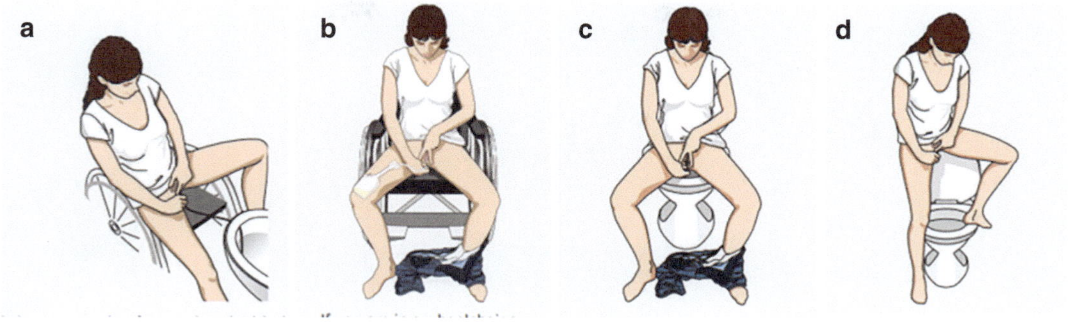

Fig. 5.3 Positions for adult females during CIC

5.4.2 Steps for Adult Females to Perform CIC

1. Wash hands with soap and running water before and after catheterization.

   Before CIC, try to touch the catheter as little as possible after washing your hands (Fig. 5.4a).

   Key points and explanations: Incorporate the learning of hand hygiene knowledge and cleaning techniques into the CIC tutorial, and emphasize that this is a simple and easy measure to avoid urinary tract infections.
2. Try to urinate on your own before catheterization, and try to expel as much urine as possible.

   Key points and explanations: Combine your own bladder function to take self-voiding, or find the "trigger point" voiding method to stimulate its reflex voiding, or use the Valsalva breath-holding method and Credé maneuver to assist voiding. This method is a non-safe voiding mode, and the use of this method needs to be guided by VUDS to ensure safety. It is forbidden for patients with high bladder pressure or VUR. Stop catheterization when the PVR after voiding is ≤100 mL.
3. Open the wet wipes and lubricant, open the catheter packaging, and tear open the packaging opening.

   Key points and explanations: At this time, do not take out the catheter.
4. Choose an appropriate position, use the left hand index finger and ring finger to separate the labia majora and minora, and at the same time, use the middle finger to lightly press the clitoris upward to expose and fix the urethral orifice (Fig. 5.4b). Beginners can seek help from family members to use a mirror and flashlight to locate the urethral orifice. After a period of practice, they can find the location of the urethral orifice by touch (Fig. 5.4c).

   Key points and instructions: When cleaning the urethral orifice and its surroundings, the direction must be from top (front) to bottom (back) to prevent the spread of bacteria and infection. The mirror should ideally have a fixed stand, with adjustable height and angle, and magnification.
5. Spray lubricant on gauze or tissue paper, and lubricate the head of the catheter.

   Key points and instructions: Strictly follow the principles of clean procedure. If conditions permit, wearing sterile gloves is a better choice. Ensure that the catheter does not touch other items. If the catheter is contaminated by touching other items, it must be replaced.
6. Place the urine collection container in a position where it can catch the urine.

   Key points and instructions: If mobility is inconvenient, for ease of procedure, the catheter can be directly connected to the urine bag.
7. Gently insert the catheter into the urethral orifice, insert it to a depth of 4–6 cm, see urine flow out, and then insert another 1 cm, to ensure it is fully inserted into the bladder (Fig. 5.4d).

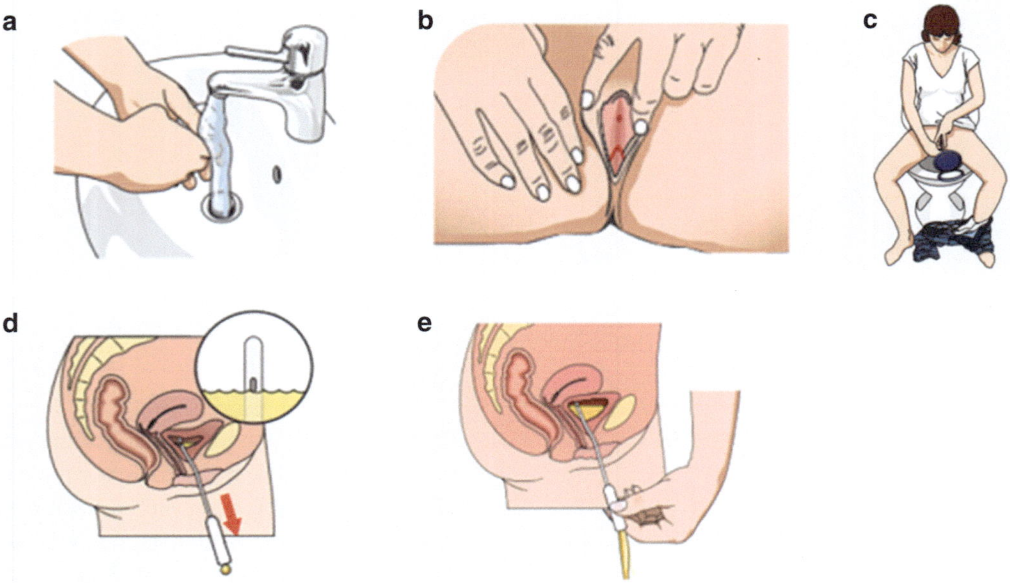

Fig. 5.4 Adult female CIC procedure

Key points and instructions: The female urethral orifice is located below the clitoris and above the vaginal opening and is wide and short. If blind insertion is used, you can first touch the clitoris with your finger and then find the urethral orifice below to prevent entry into the vagina.

8. When the urine stops flowing, slowly move the catheter, or adjust your body position. If urine flows out again, ensure that the bladder is completely emptied, and then slowly remove the catheter (Fig. 5.4e).

   Key points and instructions: When adjusting your position, you can move slightly forward and sit upright. If you are using a straight catheter, you can gently rotate the catheter and slowly pull it out. This can make the bladder empty more thoroughly. You can also apply slow pressure above the pubic bone to completely expel the urine.
9. Clean the urethral orifice with a wet tissue, and dry it with toilet paper.

   Key points and instructions: For patients who need to record urine output, use a urine pot or collection container with scales to collect urine excreted before and during catheterization, which is convenient for recording.
10. Catheterization can be performed normally during menstruation.

5.4.3 Catheter Selection for Adult Female CIC

Adult female CIC should choose a catheter of appropriate length, diameter, and head shape, which will not cause excessive pain on the one hand and can shorten the catheterization time on the other hand. Elderly women can choose hydrophilic coating and fire-polished eye catheters to reduce irritation to the urethra due to the decrease in estrogen levels.

In addition, to help female patients quickly and accurately find the urethral orifice, our team has invented two utility model patents: one is a disposable catheter with a mirror; the other is a disposable visual intermittent catheter with lighting function.

5.4.3.1 Utility Model Patent: Intermittent Catheter with Lighting Function

One end of the catheter tube of this catheter is a spherical sealing head structure, and a catheter hole is opened on the side wall of the catheter tube near the spherical sealing head. The other end of the catheter tube is equipped with a urine bag connection head. The urine bag connection head is equipped with a connection plate. The connection plate is movably equipped with a fixing plate perpendicular to the catheter tube. The fixing plate is equipped with a LED light on the side facing the spherical sealing head. The LED light is surrounded by a guide lampshade that directs the light directly to the spherical sealing head. The fixing plate is also equipped with a convex mirror above the LED light, which is used to reflect the objects at the spherical sealing head to the patient's eyes.

5.4.3.2 Utility Model Patent: Disposable Intermittent Catheter with Mirror

One end of the catheter tube of this catheter is a spherical sealing head structure, and a catheter hole is opened on the side wall of the catheter tube near the spherical sealing head. The other end of the catheter tube is equipped with a urine bag connection head. The urine bag connection head is equipped with a fixing plate perpendicular to the catheter tube. The fixing plate is facing the spherical sealing head side equipped with a convex mirror and LED light.

The difference in the structure of these two catheters gives them unique features. The catheter with lighting function concentrates light near the urethra, allowing the urethral orifice to be seen more clearly in a relatively dim environment, while the catheter with a larger mirror is more suitable for use in a relatively bright environment, making it easier to see the location of the urethral orifice. These two types of catheters are simple in structure, easy to manufacture and use, low in cost, and practical. Through the use of light sources and reflectors, they can help female patients quickly and accurately find the urethral orifice. This greatly facilitates self-catheterization operations, meeting clinical needs.

5.4.4 Considerations for Adult Female CIC

5.4.4.1 Female Psychological Characteristics Are One of the Reasons Why Female Patients Are Less Likely to Accept CIC

Studies have found that when female patients perform CIC, they feel more embarrassed than male patients. They are more resistant to CIC, especially young female patients. This may be one of the reasons for the lower acceptance level of CIC among female patients and also one of the reasons for the lower comfort level. Medical staff are the personnel who directly contact female patients, and they also play the most important role in influencing and supporting patients through the early stages. They should understand the patient's self-perception and needs, promote the establishment of patient confidence, and make CIC smoothly accepted by female patients and become a successful treatment method that can improve the quality of life. In addition, for patients who are experiencing or have experienced unpleasant lower urinary tract symptoms, CIC is more acceptable than for asymptomatic patients, because these patients believe that CIC can alleviate the troubles caused by symptoms. Therefore, before learning CIC, medical staff should be able to foresee the problem of low acceptance of CIC by female patients who have never experienced voiding dysfunction and adjust the more suitable preaching method in time. Despite the initial resistance of female patients, compared to indwelling catheters, CIC is still the best bladder management method. Patients can benefit from it, and it interferes less with daily life, improving the quality of life of female patients.

5.4.4.2 The Impact of Estrogen Changes on Adult Female CIC

Estrogen is very important for maintaining the normal function of the bladder and urethra in female patients. With age, the estrogen in women decreases year by year, especially during menopause, leading to atrophic changes in the urethral environment. These changes are related to lower urinary tract symptoms, such as frequent voiding, urgency, nocturia, incontinence, recurrent urinary tract infections, or coexisting with vaginal atrophy symptoms (such as difficulty in intercourse, itching, burning sensation, dryness, etc.). Therefore, the fear of female patients about the insertion of a catheter into sensitive areas and the worry about experiencing pain or discomfort are related to changes in body hormones and thus affect the internal environment of the urinary system. For such patients, we can choose hydrophilic-coated catheters to reduce the irritation of the catheter to the urethra.

5.4.4.3 Female Patients Who Have Had Gynecological Surgery May Need CIC

Gynecological surgery is mainly performed in the pelvic cavity. The female reproductive organs are close to the bladder and urethra, and stimulation of the bladder, urethra, and pelvic nerve plexus during surgery can affect postoperative autonomous voiding. Therefore, urinary retention is one of the common complications after gynecological surgery. The traditional treatment for urinary retention is catheterization, which can alleviate the symptoms of the patient, but it also increases the incidence of urinary tract infections and adds to the psychological burden of the patient, especially for young female patients who find it harder to accept. Moreover, postoperative catheterization is a medium-term management process, and long-term use of a catheter can easily lead to urinary system infections and other complications.

For healthy people, the bladder can regularly empty urine and has antibacterial functions. However, for patients after gynecological pelvic surgery, the bladder cannot timely and completely empty urine, causing urinary retention. Its defense function drops sharply, making it more susceptible to external pathogen infections, increasing the risk of infection, and easily causing urinary tract infections. CIC can continuously enhance the autonomous voiding ability of the bladder in patients with urinary retention after gynecological surgery, gradually restoring its normal physiological functions and also freeing the patient from the catheter, which plays an important role in the recovery of postoperative autonomous voiding function and physical and mental health.

5.5 Adult Male CIC Techniques

Compared to female patients, due to the different anatomy of the urethra, the actual procedure and precautions of CIC in male are slightly different.

5.5.1 Characteristics of the Male Urethra

We have already detailed the anatomical structure of the male and female urethra. Compared to females, the male urethra is long and curved. How to correctly identify indications, combined with the anatomical characteristics of the male urethra to perform CIC, is a key technique that health-care worker and patients and their families who perform CIC need to master.

The male urethra starts at the internal urethral orifice and ends at the external urethral orifice at the tip of the penis. It is 17–20 cm long in adults and can be divided into three parts: the prostatic part (the part that passes through the prostate), the membranous part (the part that passes through the urogenital diaphragm, about 1.2 cm), and the spongy part (the part that passes through the urethral sponge); clinically, the prostate part and the membranous part are collectively referred to as the posterior urethra, and the spongy part is referred to as the anterior urethra. The male urethra varies in thickness during its course, with three narrowings, three dilations, and two bends. The three narrowings are located at the internal orifice of the urethra, the membranous part, and the external orifice of the urethra. The two bends are the anterior pubic bend and the inferior pubic bend. When performing CIC procedures, these anatomical features of the male urethra should be kept in mind to avoid damaging the urethra.

Apart from patients with phimosis or hypospadias, the external orifice of the male urethra is mostly easy to locate, but the male urethra is long and has three narrow parts and two bends, which adds certain difficulties to CIC, and it requires training and practice to master it proficiently.

5.5.2 Main Steps of Male CIC

Choose a comfortable and clean environment and position. It can be done in the bathroom, shower room, wheelchair, bed at home or accessible bathrooms, cubicles, at workplace/school, etc.

5.5.2.1 Prepare Supplies

1. Choose the appropriate catheter size and type: 14–16 Fr is the most commonly used diameter size for adult males. If unsure about the size, always start with a smaller diameter, and increase the size as needed. Patients who have difficulty passing a regular catheter due to urethral narrowing or obstruction can choose a Coudé catheter with a curved tip. This catheter is particularly useful for patients with BPH or elevated bladder neck.
2. Prepare a urine collection container, preferably a graduated container, to measure the amount of urine drained, such as a measuring cup, etc.
3. Prepare cleaning agents and towels, or open wet wipes and lubricants. Open the catheter, and just tear open the packaging opening.

   Key points and explanations: At this time, do not take out the catheter. Strictly implement the principle of no-touch technique procedure. For male patients who are sensitive to pain, it is recommended to use a local anesthetic gel or emulsion analgesic.
4. Prepare gloves (without latex components) if possible.
5. Prepare consumables on a clean table. Place the prepared catheter on a clean table; if it is a hydrophilic catheter, add water to the catheter packaging, or break the water bag containing the catheter; if it is a regular catheter, evenly apply lubricating gel to cover the entire catheter surface.
6. Place the drainage container in a position where it can catch the urine.

   Key points and instructions: If the mobility is inconvenient, to facilitate procedure, the catheter can be connected to a urine collection bag.

5.5.2.2 If Possible, Try to Urinate on Your Own Before Inserting the Catheter

Key points and instructions: Depending on your own bladder function, you can either self-urinate or find a "trigger point" to stimulate reflexive voiding, or use the Valsalva breath-holding method and Credé maneuver to assist voiding. This method is not a safe voiding mode, and its use should be guided by VUDS to ensure safety. It is contraindicated for patients with high bladder pressure and vesicoureteral reflux.

5.5.2.3 Choose the Appropriate Position

The position for catheterization can be standing (Fig. 5.5a); sitting on the toilet or wheelchair (Fig. 5.5b–d); or sitting or lying on your side.

5.5.2.4 Perform Hand Hygiene

Clean both hands; generally, wash hands with soap and running water (Fig. 5.6a).

Key points and instructions: It is recommended to use the seven-step hand washing method. If conditions do not allow, you can also directly use quick hand sanitizer.

5.5.2.5 CIC Procedure

1. One hand holds the penis and pushes the foreskin back to expose the urethral orifice, while the other hand takes a disposable wet wipe to clean the urethral orifice, glans, coronal sulcus, and root of the penis in turn. Each cleaning tissue or cotton pad can only be used once; please do not reuse. Pay attention to fully expose the procedure area, men who have not undergone circumcision should turn over the foreskin, expose the urethral orifice, and then clean; if conditions permit, sterile gloves can be worn for procedure. For patients with bladder stoma, use soap and clean water or non-irritating odor disinfectant to wipe and clean the stoma and surrounding area.
2. Open the wet wipes and lubricant. Open the catheter, and just tear open the packaging opening.

   Key points and instructions: At this time, do not take out the catheter. Strictly implement the principle of no-touch technique procedure. For male patients who are sensitive to pain, it is recommended to use local anesthetic gel or emulsion analgesic.
3. Spray the lubricant on a gauze or paper towel, pinch the package to pick up the catheter, and lubricate the catheter with the paper towel.

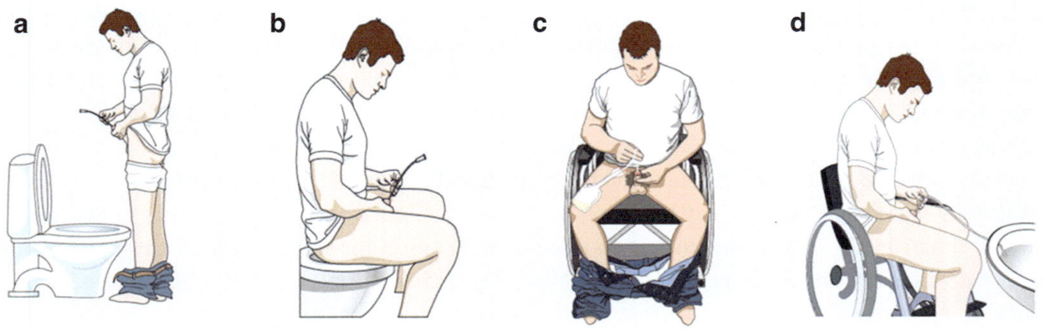

Fig. 5.5 Male CIC position

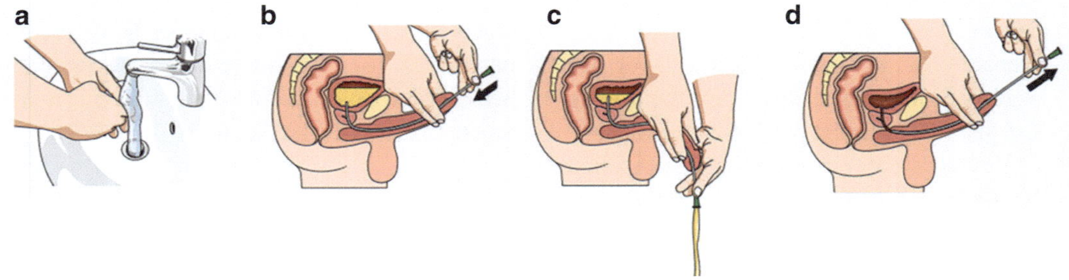

Fig. 5.6 Male CIC procedure steps

Key points and instructions: Make sure your hand does not touch the end of the catheter to be inserted and does not touch other objects and other parts of the body. If the catheter is contaminated, it must be replaced.

4. Hold the penis with one hand, and lift it up, making it a 60° angle with the abdominal wall to eliminate the anterior pubic curvature (Fig. 5.6b). Take out the catheter with the other hand, and perform the catheterization procedure. After the catheter passes through the first urethral bend, bend the penis down, and continue to insert the catheter (Fig. 5.6c). Generally, insert into the urethra 17–20 cm.

   Key points and instructions: Do not grip the penis tightly, and relax your body at the same time to avoid resistance to the insertion of the catheter. The action of catheterization should be gentle. The male urethra has three narrowings, so avoid using too much force too quickly to damage the urethral mucosa. If insertion is difficult, you can pause for a while, take deep breaths at the same time, appropriately change the insertion angle, and avoid repeated pulling and inserting to cause urethral injury. If the catheter cannot pass, try to reposition the penis. If unsuccessful, do not force it.

5. When the catheter is inserted into the bladder, urine can be seen flowing out. At this time, the catheter should be pushed into the bladder another 1–2 cm, and continue to drain until the bladder is emptied; when the urine stops flowing out, adjust the body position such as moving forward and sitting straight to ensure that the bladder is completely emptied.
6. After the urine is drained, slowly pull out the catheter. When half of it is pulled out, tilt the penis upward, and pull out the entire catheter (Fig. 5.6d). If urine flows out when the catheter is pulled out, please pause the removal of the catheter, and let the urine completely drain out.

Key points and instructions: If you are using a straight catheter, you can gently rotate the catheter and slowly pull it out, which can make the bladder empty more thoroughly, and you can also slowly apply pressure on the pubic bone to completely drain the urine.

7. After the catheter is removed, clean the urethral orifice with a wet paper towel, and restore the foreskin to its original position. Wash your hands.

   Key points and instructions: For patients who need to record urine output, you can collect the urine that is excreted before catheterization and the urine that is excreted during catheterization with a scaled urine pot or urine collection container, and record it in the voiding diary.
8. Clean your hands.

5.5.3 Precautions for Male CIC

The implementation of continuous catheterization can be performed by medical personnel, and the procedure is relatively simple; while CIC procedure requires the patient or family members to operate themselves, there is a certain training period, and the male urethra is longer than the female, and the catheterization is more difficult in male than that of female patients. Therefore, paying more attention is needed to the contraindications of CIC, including urethral stricture, false passage in the urethra, small bladder, or contracted bladder.

For men performing CIC, in addition to paying attention to hand hygiene and catheter cleanliness, it is more important to understand the anatomical structure of the male urethra and teach them the method of catheterization, and it is recommended to use the front-end curved Coudé catheter (Fig. 5.7). The Coudé catheter has a curved tip and is used for patients who have difficulty passing through a straight catheter due to urethral stricture or obstruction. The Coudé catheter is particularly useful for patients with BPH or elevated bladder neck. The curved part faces the ventral side of the penis, closely entering the anterior wall of the urethra until the catheter is fully inserted into the urethra and urine flows out.

Patients undergoing bladder expansion surgery may need bladder irrigation and a larger size of catheter due to mucus production. Before catheterization, lubricate the entire catheter with a

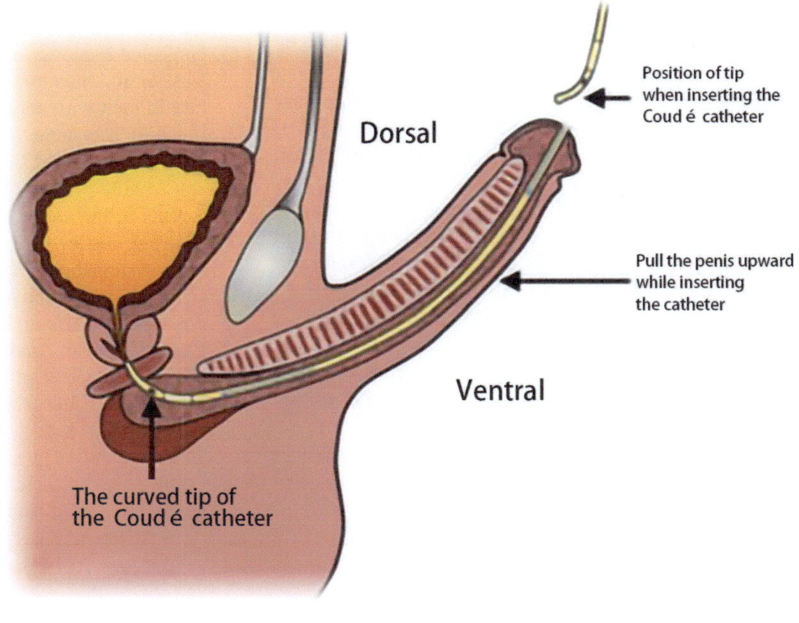

Fig. 5.7 The front-end curved Coudé catheter is used for catheterization in BPH patients; note that the direction of the catheter head is toward the abdomen

sufficient amount of lubricant to avoid dryness causing patient pain and urethral mucosal injury. After the failure of catheter retention, do not repeatedly attempt multiple times, and seek help from health-care worker in time. During CIC, pay attention to the patient's reaction; some patients may feel dizzy and/or faint after suddenly draining a large amount of urine.

The frequency of CIC is generally once every 4 hours on average or 300–400 mL each time, but it may vary. The doctor will determine the frequency. Also, the use of sterile gloves is encouraged during CIC.

In summary, adult male CIC should pay attention to indications and contraindications and pay attention to the anatomical characteristics of the male urethra during the procedure. Long-term CIC patients should pay attention to regular kidney and bladder function and morphology assessment, especially urodynamic assessment, understand the safe capacity of the bladder, and adjust the number and time of CIC in time.

References

1. Dinh A, Davido B, Duran C, et al. Urinary tract infections in patients with neurogenic bladder [J]. Med Mal Infect. 2019;49(7):495–504. https://doi.org/10.1016/j.medmal.2019.02.006.
2. Fuentes M, Magalhães J, Barroso U Jr. Diagnosis and management of bladder dysfunction in neurologically normal children [J]. Front Pediatr. 2019;7:298.
3. Groen J, Pannek J, Castro Diaz D, et al. Summary of European Association of Urology (EAU) guidelines on neuro-urology [J]. Eur Urol. 2016;69(2):324–33.
4. Yang SS, Chiang IN, Lin CD, Chang SJ. Advances in non-surgical treatments for urinary tract infections in children [J]. World J Urol. 2012;30(1):69–75. https://doi.org/10.1007/s00345-011-0700-5.
5. Sager C, Barroso U Jr, Bastos JMN, et al. Management of neurogenic bladder dysfunction in children update and recommendations on medical treatment [J]. Int Braz J Urol. 2022;48(1):31–51. https://doi.org/10.1590/s1677-5538.Ibju.2020.0989.
6. Newman DK, Willson MM. Review of intermittent catheterization and current best practices [J]. Urol Nurs. 2011;31(1):12–28, 48; quiz 29.
7. Wyndaele JJ, Brauner A, Geerlings SE, et al. Clean intermittent catheterization and urinary tract infection: review and guide for future research [J]. BJU Int. 2012;110(11 Pt C):E910–7. https://doi.org/10.1111/j.1464-410X.2012.11549.x.
8. Mcmonnies G. Paediatric continence in children with neuropathic bladders [J]. Br J Nurs. 2002;11(11):765–72. https://doi.org/10.12968/bjon.2002.11.11.765.
9. Sand PK, Sand RI. The diagnosis and management of lower urinary tract symptoms in multiple sclerosis patients [J]. Dis Mon. 2013;59(7):261–8. https://doi.org/10.1016/j.disamonth.2013.03.013.
10. De Jong TP, Chrzan R, Klijn AJ, Dik P. Treatment of the neurogenic bladder in spina bifida [J]. Pediatr Nephrol. 2008;23(6):889–96. https://doi.org/10.1007/s00467-008-0780-7.
11. Herbert AS, Welk B, Elliott CS. Internal and external barriers to bladder management in persons with neurologic disease performing intermittent catheterization [J]. Int J Environ Res Public Health. 2023;20(12):6079. https://doi.org/10.3390/ijerph20126079.
12. Malde S, Belal M, Mohamed-Ahmed R, et al. Can we define the optimal postvoid residual volume at which intermittent catheterization should be recommended, and are there other measures that could guide an intermittent catheterization protocol: ICI-RS 2023 [J]. Neurourol Urodyn. 2023;43:1353. https://doi.org/10.1002/nau.25324.
13. Stein R, Bogaert G, Dogan HS, et al. EAU/ESPU guidelines on the management of neurogenic bladder in children and adolescent part II operative management [J]. Neurourol Urodyn. 2020;39(2):498–506. https://doi.org/10.1002/nau.24248.
14. Cendron M, Gearhart JP. The Mitrofanoff principle. Technique and application in continent urinary diversion [J]. Urol Clin North Am. 1991;18(4):615–21.
15. González-Espinosa C, Castro-Nuñez P, Averbeck MA, et al. Diagnosis and treatment of urethral stricture in men with neurogenic lower urinary tract dysfunction: a systematic review [J]. Neurourol Urodyn. 2022;41(6):1248–57. https://doi.org/10.1002/nau.24982.
16. Çetinel B, Tarcan T, Demirkesen O, et al. Management of lower urinary tract dysfunction in multiple sclerosis: a systematic review and Turkish consensus report [J]. Neurourol Urodyn. 2013;32(8):1047–57. https://doi.org/10.1002/nau.22374.
17. Kurtz MJ, Van Zandt DK, Sapp LR. A new technique in independent intermittent catheterization: the Mitrofanoff catheterizable channel [J]. Rehabil Nurs. 1996;21(6):311–4. https://doi.org/10.1002/j.2048-7940.1996.tb01353.x.
18. Elliott CS, Dallas K, Shem K, Crew J. Adoption of single-use clean intermittent catheterization poli-

cies does not appear to affect genitourinary outcomes in a large spinal cord injury cohort [J]. J Urol. 2022;208(5):1055–74.
19. Chu DI, Kayle M, Stern A, et al. Longitudinal trajectories of clean intermittent catheterization responsibility in youths with spina bifida [J]. J Urol. 2022;207(1):192–200.
20. Balhi S, Arfaouni RB, Mrabet A. Intermittent catheterisation: the common complications [J]. Br J Community Nurs. 2021;26(6):272–7.
21. Kidd EA, Stewart F, Kassis NC, et al. Urethral (indwelling or intermittent) or suprapubic routes for short-term catheterisation in hospitalised adults [J]. Cochrane Database Syst Rev. 2015;2015(12):CD004203. https://doi.org/10.1002/14651858.CD004203.pub3.

6 Characteristics of Pediatric CIC

Jian-Guo Wen

The treatment principle of pediatric NB is to prevent VUR and hydronephrosis, prevent upper urinary tract injury, and protect kidney function. Therefore, timely emptying of the bladder and maintaining a low-pressure state bladder is particularly important for the treatment of NB children, which is the key to preventing VUR and hydronephrosis and other upper urinary tract damage. For NB children who cannot empty their bladder on their own, a catheter can be retained, or CIC can be used to assist in emptying the bladder.

CIC regular drainage of urine can reduce the pressure in the bladder, prevent the increase of PVR in the bladder, keep the bladder content below the safe capacity, maintain a low pressure state in the bladder, prevent VUR and hydronephrosis, prevent upper urinary tract injury, protect renal function, and improve the quality of life. Although CIC has been considered as a first-line treatment for NB internationally, there are still few long-term follow-up studies on the effect of CIC treatment on NB. In addition, there is still controversy about when to start CIC for NB patients and whether to start CIC as soon as the diagnosis is clear. The author provides a reference for the implementation of CIC in clinical practice by systematically discussing the indications, contraindications, procedure, and characteristics of children's CIC compared to adults.

J.-G. Wen (✉)
Pediatric Urodynamic Center/Department of Urology, First Affiliated Hospital of Zhengzhou University, Zhengzhou, China

6.1 Indications and Contraindications for CIC in Children [1]

CIC is applicable to various neurogenic and non-neurogenic factors causing bladder emptying disorders, such as congenital spinal cord maldevelopment, meningitis, cerebral palsy, or pelvic diseases in children causing neurological dysfunction leading to detrusor non-function or low activity, leading to BOO, causing detrusor compensatory hyperplasia and fibrosis, filling incontinence caused by detrusor non-contraction, urgency incontinence caused by overactive detrusor, bladder emptying disorder caused by excessive inhibition of reflex hyperactive detrusor by anticholinergic drugs, increased PVR, post bladder augmentation, and voiding disorder caused by NB. All of the above situations can use CIC to assist in emptying the bladder and protecting the upper urinary tract. But CIC is contraindicated in children with the following conditions: urinary system malformation, severe urethritis, cystitis, urethral bleeding, urethral stricture, perineal abscess, and inconvenient movement of both upper limbs.

J.-G. Wen (ed.), *Progress in Clean Intermittent Catheterization*, Experts' Perspectives on Medical Advances, https://doi.org/10.1007/978-981-97-5021-4_6

The application of CIC in adult patients is very widespread, with literature reporting that about 56% of NB patients in the United States choose CIC to treat bladder dysfunction, and patients need to perform CIC for a long time or for life. The application of CIC in pediatric NB is not as widespread as in adults, and there is still controversy about when to perform CIC for NB patients and under what circumstances to start CIC. Some foreign scholars believe that if the physical examination of the patient is negative and there is no hydronephrosis, it is not recommended to perform CIC until clinical manifestations such as UTI or hydronephrosis appear, and then UDS is performed to determine whether to start CIC. They believe that it is not feasible to let all NB patients perform CIC early, and treatment based on clinical manifestations is sufficient to protect upper urinary tract function. Even if CIC is not performed early, UDS should be performed earlier to ensure high-risk patients should undergo CIC if they exhibit increased leakage point pressure, detrusor-sphincter dyssynergia (DSD), or decreased bladder compliance (BC) [2]. Some experts believe that children should start CIC in infancy, giving parents and the child ample time to adapt to this bladder management method, which helps to maintain a moderate bladder wall thickness and increase bladder compliance. Early CIC in children is crucial for preventing renal damage and bladder dysfunction and reducing the chance of future surgeries. Some believe that if urodynamic studies during follow-up show the bladder is in a safe state, CIC should be stopped. However, others support continuing CIC, arguing that most children will need to continue CIC to achieve urinary bladder control, and if the child is already accustomed to CIC, this goal is more easily achieved [3].

6.2 Choice of CIC Catheter for Children

Whether a child can persist with CIC long term is greatly related to the convenience and ease of use of the catheter. These factors include ease of unpacking, easy grip of the catheter, easy insertion, less friction during insertion and removal, fewer steps in the process, easy portability of the catheter, and no need for cleaning [4]. Additionally, parents prefer catheters that achieve the best results, such as reducing friction and trauma to the urethra, lowering the incidence of urethral and urinary adhesions, and reducing the frequency of urinary system infections. Therefore, choosing a suitable or high-quality CIC catheter becomes particularly important. In recent years, with the advancement of technology, CIC catheters have seen significant improvements around the above performance indicators and are gradually being promoted in clinical practice, achieving good clinical results.

6.2.1 Material of Children's CIC Catheter

Studies have shown that children's compliance with hydrophilic-coated catheters is higher than with regular catheters [5]. Compared to regular PVC catheters, children prefer using hydrophilic-coated catheters because they have less friction, lower incidence of urethral and urinary adhesions, reduced UTI rates, and improved patient compliance. Additionally, there are antibiotic-coated catheters, which have antibiotics applied to their surface, but children may be allergic to this, or it could lead to the emergence of superbugs. Due to the small and delicate nature of a child's urethra, it is necessary to choose a hydrophilic-coated catheter that can reduce urethral friction, decrease trauma and adhesions, and reduce symptomatic UTIs. This makes it more tolerable for the children and helps to reduce the difficulty of pediatric CIC, and the reduction in urethral injury and other complications also makes it easier for parents and children to accept long-term treatment.

If a non-hydrophilic-coated catheter is used, a lubricant should be applied to the surface of the catheter to reduce urethral friction [6]. Clinically, water-soluble lubricants and paraffin oil lubricants are commonly used. However, because water-soluble lubricants have good biocompatibility, are easily absorbed by the body, do not remain in the body for a long time, have small toxic side effects, and have better lubrication, it is better to use water-soluble lubricants. Considering the cost of the catheter and the family conditions of the patient, the choice of catheter can vary from person to person, referring to the following standards: the catheter is smooth and comfortable to use and can be easily inserted into the urethra, and the procedure is simple when catheterizing. Choose the catheter with the highest cost-effectiveness for the children under economically permissible conditions.

6.2.2 Size and Tip of the Catheter

Choosing the right size catheter is key to successful catheterization in children [7]. The development of modern technology has made it possible to manufacture catheters of various sizes needed in clinical practice. Children generally choose 6–12 Fr catheters, and the specific size is adjusted according to the individual, to avoid too big catheters damaging the urethral mucosa of infants and young children and also to avoid too thin catheters being blocked. If there is no suitable size catheter for infants, a suitable nasogastric tube can be used instead. The urethra of children is shorter than that of adults, so there is no need to use too long catheters, to avoid the catheter bending in the bladder, affecting the discharge of urine; short catheters are convenient to use, and the requirements for the length of the catheter vary depending on the catheterization environment in actual application [8].

Because the female urethra is short and straight, short catheters are just suitable for the physiological structure of the female urethra, so the catheters chosen by female patients can be shorter than boys. Urine is discharged through the holes on the catheter; the larger the size of the catheter, the larger the corresponding holes, and the drainage holes made by hot melt technology are smoother than cold punched holes. Different types of catheter tips meet the needs of different patients. The straight tip catheter is suitable for most children, its pointed design allows it to be smoothly inserted into the urethra, and urine enters the tube cavity through the two holes on the catheter; the bent head catheter has a curved tube head, designed with one to three drainage holes, suitable for children with narrow urethra; the soft round head catheter can prevent damage caused by the catheter passing through the urethra, suitable for all patients.

6.2.3 How Long Is the Catheter Used

The most widely used at present is the disposable catheter, not reused. Ordinary reusable catheters can also be used, but these catheters are not as convenient to carry and use as disposable ones. After each use, it needs to be sterilized by boiling or soaking in disinfectant. If the catheter is damaged or blocked, it should be replaced in time, and the use time should not exceed 1 week. The specific choice of which type of catheter can be determined according to the economic conditions of the child's family, but no matter which type is chosen, the quality and safety of the catheter must be ensured.

6.3 Procedure of CIC for Children

6.3.1 Preparation

The doctor explains to the parents and children the progression and treatment methods of NB disease, informs them of the purpose and efficacy of CIC, eliminates the fear of catheterization in the children and their parents, prepares them for long-term catheterization, selects the appropriate catheter, and ensures the comfort of the child as much as possible. The doctor demonstrates to the parents and the children how to catheterize correctly, explains the drinking plan and interval time, and informs them of the precautions. For infants and young children who cannot catheterize themselves, the parents replace the children in learning and assist the children in catheterization. When the children reach school age, the parents should gradually let the children learn to catheterize themselves so that they can operate on their own at school.

6.3.2 Procedure

Before CIC, clean your hands, and maintain the hygiene of the genitals, and wash at least twice a day, preferably before the child catheterizes. Fully expose the urethral orifice, keep the field of vision clear, infants and young children can take the supine or sitting position, older children can also stand or squat, and adopt the most suitable posture according to individual circumstances. The anatomy of the child's urinary system is slightly different from that of adults, its bladder position is higher, the newborn's bladder is often located above the pubic symphysis, it is pear-shaped, and the infant's bladder is closer to the anterior abdominal wall and gradually descends with age. It descends into the pelvic cavity. The normal boy's urethra is 5–6 cm long at 1 year old and about 12 cm at puberty; the girl's urethra is shorter than the boy's, only 1 cm after birth, and can grow to 2–3 cm later. The urethral orifice of the male child patient is obvious, the thumb and index finger hold the catheter, and slowly insert it into the urethra. When inserting the catheter, lift the penis toward the abdominal side to straighten the urethra, and avoid injuring the urethral isthmus. The female child patient's urethra is more hidden, located between the clitoris and the vagina, parents should assist during CIC, and be careful to find it to avoid inserting catheter into the vagina. Older female patients can use a mirror to find the urethra when catheterizing themselves. The female urethra is shorter than the male's, so the insertion length should also be shorter than the male's to avoid the catheter knotting in the bladder. The male child patient needs to pass the front end of the catheter beyond the internal orifice of the urethra, see urine flowing out, and then insert the catheter further into the urethra 1–2 cm. While female infants can first insert the catheter about 1.5 cm into the urethra, after urine flows out, insert it further about 0.5 cm, and the specific length can be determined according to the age of the child patient. Check whether the flowing urine is turbid and whether the color is abnormal. Avoid squeezing the bladder with your hand when the urine just flows out to prevent VUR. During the urine flow, keep the catheter opening facing down. When the urine flow becomes thin, you can rotate the catheter at multiple angles to change the position of the side holes, and insert or withdraw the catheter a little from the bladder. After the urine flow stops, you can increase the abdominal pressure or lightly press on the pubic bone with your hand. This helps to squeeze out the PVR, and then slowly pull out the catheter. If urine flows out during the process, pause for a moment until all the urine has flowed out, and then completely remove the catheter. When removing the catheter, make sure the catheter is lower than the level of the urethra (Fig. 6.1). Be careful not to forcefully insert the catheter. If insertion is not smooth, you can apply more lubricant and try again. If insertion is still difficult, seek help from a doctor.

6.3.2.1 Steps for Male Children's CIC

1. Choose the position according to the boy's age or specific situation.

   Position 1: supine position, suitable for newborns or infants.

   Position 2: lying on the side of the bed, suitable for older children.

   Position 3: sitting in a wheelchair, suitable for older children who cannot stand.

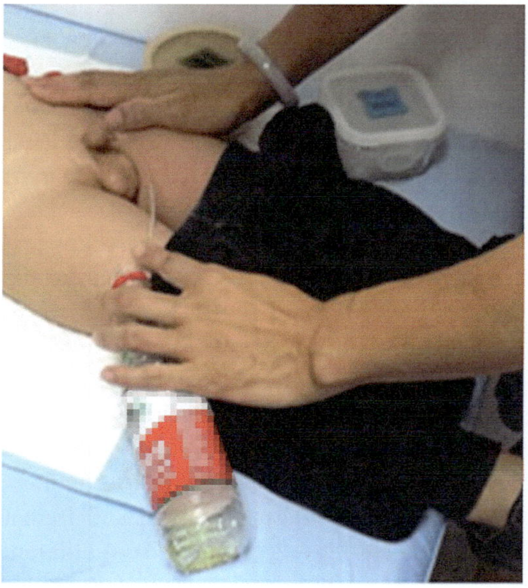

Fig. 6.1 Parents assisting a 3-year-old patient with CIC, and urine is being exported (see color insert 4)

Position 4: sitting on the toilet or sitting on the bed with knees bent outward, suitable for older children.

Position 5: standing position, suitable for older children.

2. Prepare all items in the order of catheterization, placed in a convenient location (Fig. 6.2).

   Key points and explanations: Encourage children to prepare items and operate on their own. Initially, catheterization can be performed with the help of dedicated health-care worker or parents, gradually cultivating the child's ability to operate independently.

3. Try to urinate on your own, but don't strain too hard.

   Wash and dry your hands with soap and running water, and keep your nails short and clean (Figs. 6.3 and 6.4).

   Key points and explanations: It is recommended to use the seven-step hand washing method.

4. Stand in front of the toilet, sit on a chair straddling the toilet, or lie flat or on your side on the bed.
5. For children with phimosis, the foreskin should be pulled back and kept in place during catheterization, exposing the urinary meatus. Clean the penis and urinary meatus with clean water or a wet wipe (Figs. 6.5 and 6.6).
6. Apply lubricant to the front end of the catheter. It should cover the front 6–8 cm of the catheter. Tips and instructions: Beginners are recommended to use a suitable hydrophilic-coated catheter. It is suggested that those with sensitive urethra use lidocaine cream for local anesthesia to reduce pain and discomfort.
7. Hold the penis with one hand, and lift it toward the abdominal wall to expose the urinary meatus. Hold the catheter with the another hand like grasping a pencil, and slowly insert it into the urethra 6–12 cm, and insert another 1–2 cm when urine flows out (Figs. 6.7 and 6.8).

   Tips and instructions: High mental tension can cause increased resistance in the urethral sphincter, and instruct the children to breathe slowly and deeply, which helps with the insertion of the catheter. Avoid contaminating the catheter during the insertion process.

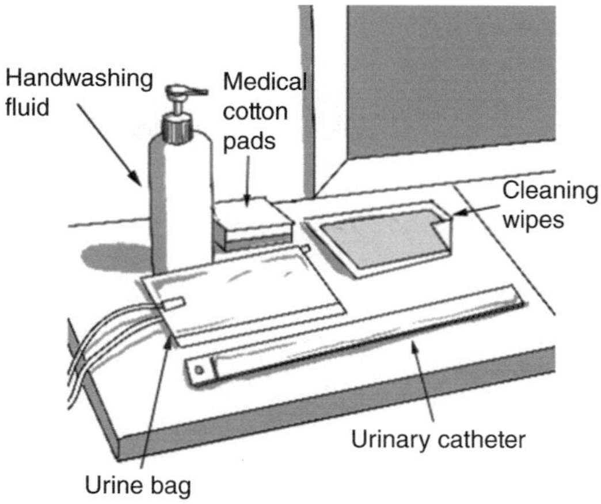

Fig. 6.2 Items placed in a convenient location. (Drawn by Li Qingpeng, Yanshan University, Class of 2016)

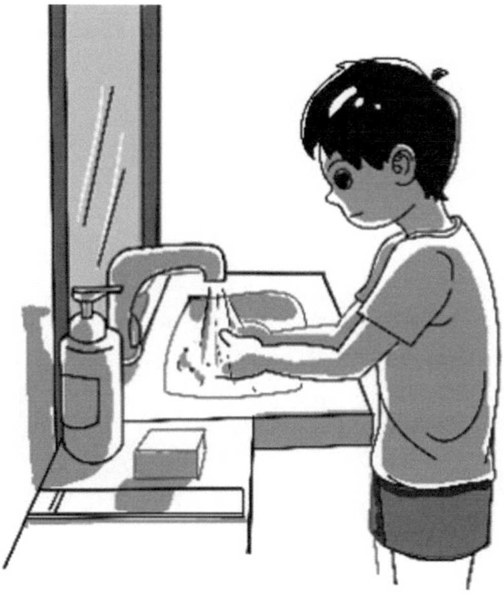

Fig. 6.3 Washing hands while standing. (Drawn by Li Qingpeng)

8. Drain the urine into the toilet or a urine collection container.

   Key points and explanations: For children who need to record urine output, a graduated urinal or urine collection container can be used to collect the urine excreted before and during catheterization, which is convenient for recording.

9. When voiding stops, slowly remove the catheter. Urine will still flow out and continue to be excreted until no more urine flows out.

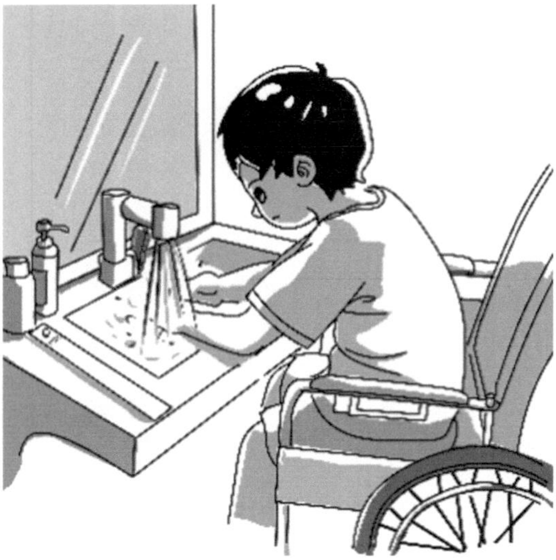

Fig. 6.4 A boy with mobility difficulties washing his hands while sitting in a wheelchair. (Drawn by Li Qingpeng)

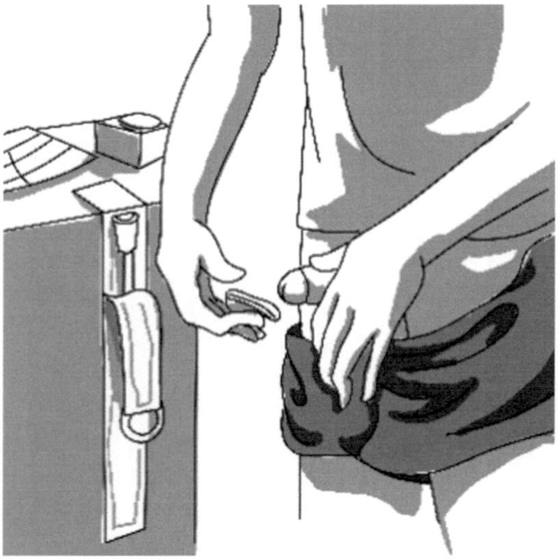

Fig. 6.5 Washing the penis and urinary meatus while standing. (Drawn by Li Qingpeng)

Key points and explanations: When adjusting the position, you can move slightly forward and sit upright, and if you are using a straight catheter, you can slowly pull it out while gently rotating the catheter, which can make the bladder empty more thoroughly. Wipe the penis clean, reposition the foreskin, and wash your hands.

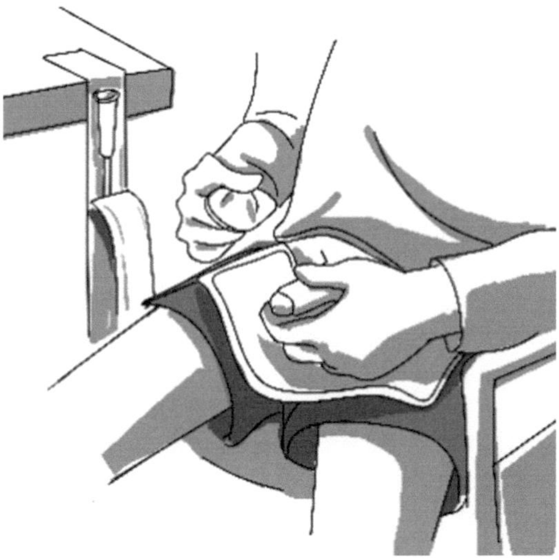

Fig. 6.6 A boy with mobility difficulties washing his penis and urinary meatus while sitting in a wheelchair

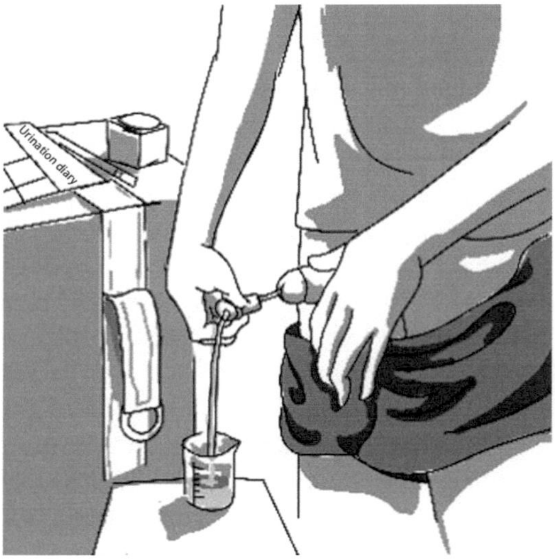

Fig. 6.7 Inserting the catheter while standing

Key points and explanations: Due to the special nature of the area involved in catheterization, and children are in the growth development stage, the awareness of sexual protection is weak; parents or caregivers should pay special attention to protecting the privacy and safety of children, to prevent psychological trauma to minors or even violation. Organize catheterization supplies; catheterization ends.

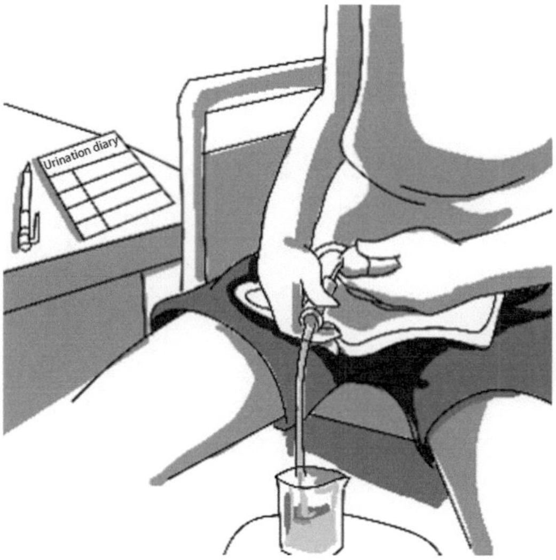

Fig. 6.8 Inserting a catheter while sitting in a wheelchair

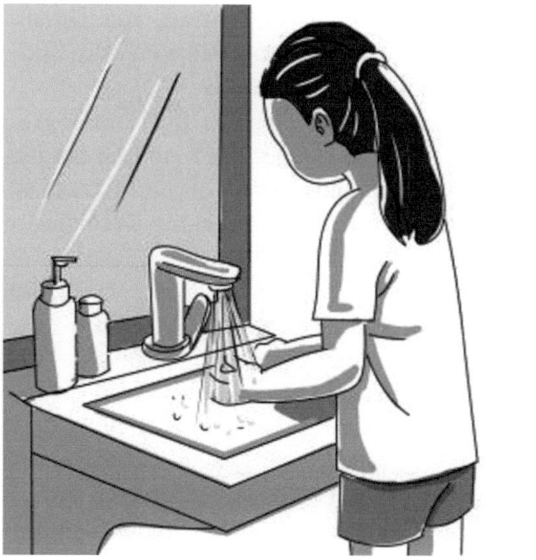

Fig. 6.9 Washing hands in standing position. (Illustrated by Li Qingpeng)

6.3.2.2 Female Children CIC Procedure Steps

1. Position

   Position 1: Sit in a wheelchair, with both feet on the toilet seat.

   Position 2: Sit in a wheelchair, lift one foot onto the wheelchair cushion.

   Position 3: Semi-recumbent position, both legs bent outward.

   Position 4: Sit on the toilet, with both feet on the footrest.

   Position 5: Squat on the squat toilet.

   Position 6: Stand, with one foot lifted onto the toilet seat.

2. Prepare all items, and put them together in a place that is easy to reach (same as the preparation of CIC items for boys).

   Key points and explanations: Encourage children to prepare items and operate on their own. Initially, catheterization can be done with the help of parents or caregivers, gradually cultivating the child's ability to operate independently.

3. First urinate on your own, no need to push too hard.
4. Wash and dry your hands with soap and water, and keep your nails short and clean (Figs. 6.9 and 6.10).

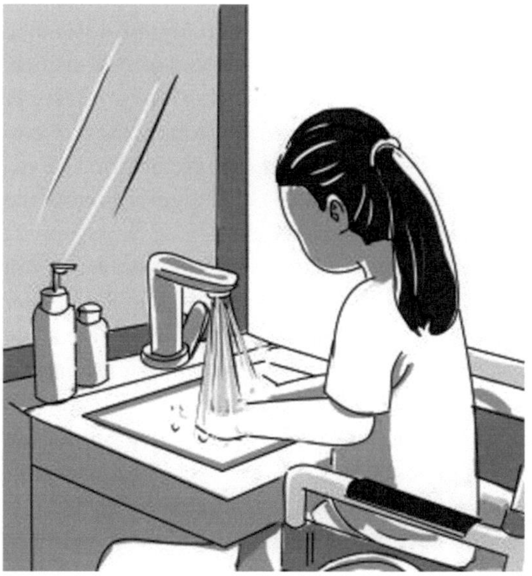

Fig. 6.10 A girl with mobility difficulties washing her hands while sitting in a wheelchair. (Illustrated by Li Qingpeng)

   Key points and explanations: It is recommended to use the seven-step hand washing method.

5. Ensure a comfortable posture. You can sit on the toilet or on a chair straddling the toilet,

with your feet on the footrest. You can also stand, with one leg propped on the edge of the chair or toilet.

Use one hand to separate the labia (vaginal folds) and the another hand to clean the urethral orifice and surrounding area from top (front) to bottom (back) with a wet wipe, or use a small mirror for cleaning (Fig. 6.11).

Key points and instructions: To prevent slipping, you can wrap dry gauze or tissue around your thumb and index finger.

6. Apply lubricant to the front end of the catheter. It should cover the last 5–8 cm of the catheter. Touch your clitoris with one finger, and use a light source and a mirror to help find the correct position of the urethral orifice. Occasionally inserting the catheter into the vagina is a normal phenomenon.

   Key points and instructions: Choose a catheter of the right size and material.
7. Use the thumb and index finger of your left hand to spread the labia to the sides and upward, fully exposing the urethral orifice. With the help of a mirror, slowly insert the lubricated catheter into the urethra 4–5 cm; when urine flows out, insert another 1–2 cm (Figs. 6.12 and 6.13). Then gently move the catheter 3 cm further away.

   Key points and instructions: The sphincter will have some resistance, like a door in the bladder neck. It is important to slow down your breathing and relax your muscles. Avoid contaminating the catheter during the insertion process.
8. All urine is drained into the toilet or container.

   Key points and explanations: For patients who need to record urine volume, a urine pot or urine collection container with scales can be used to collect the urine that is excreted on their own before catheterization and the urine that is excreted during catheterization, which is convenient for recording.
9. When voiding stops, slowly remove the catheter. Urine will still flow out and continue to be excreted until no more urine flows out.

   Key points and explanations: When adjusting the position, you can move slightly forward and sit upright, and if you are using a straight catheter, you can gently rotate the catheter and slowly pull it out, which can make the bladder empty more thoroughly.

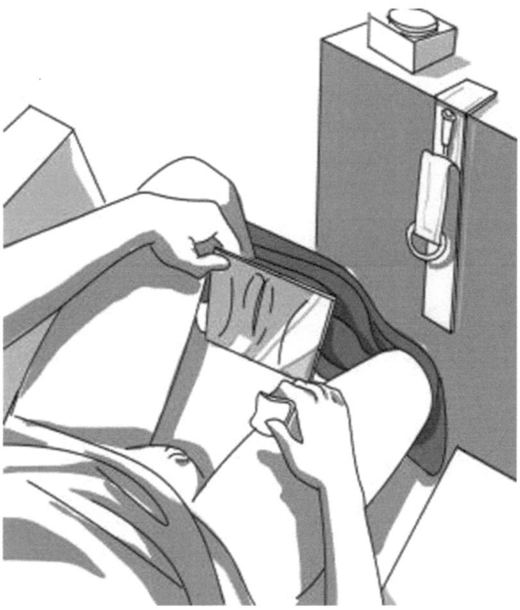

Fig. 6.11 Cleaning the perineum with the help of a small mirror. (Illustrated by Li Qingpeng)

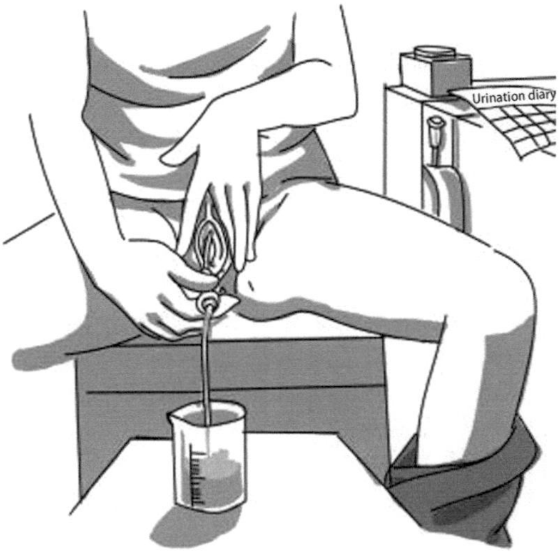

Fig. 6.12 A girl sitting on a stool inserting a catheter with her right hand. (Illustrated by Li Qingpeng)

Let the children wipe the perineum clean and wash their hands.

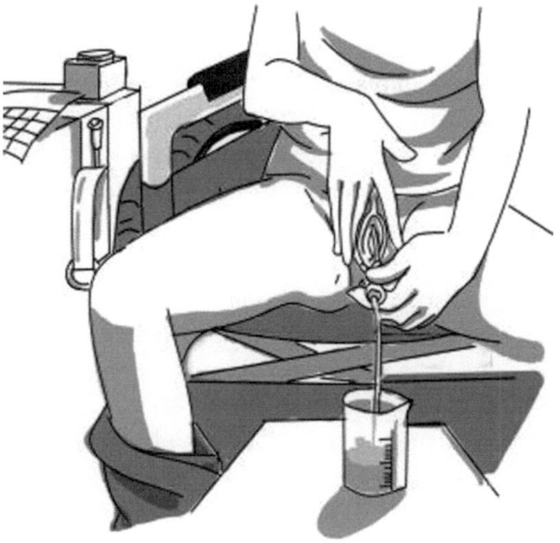

Fig. 6.13 Girl inserting a catheter with her left hand. (Drawn by Li Qingpeng)

Key points and explanations: Due to the special nature of the area involved in catheterization, children are in the growth and development stage, their awareness of sexual protection is weak, and parents or caregivers should pay special attention to protecting the children's privacy and safety to prevent psychological trauma to minors or even violation.

Organize catheterization supplies; catheterization ends.

6.3.3 Frequency of Children's CIC

The frequency of CIC is crucial to the treatment effect of the patients. Too few catheterizations may cause the bacteria in the urine to stay in the bladder for a long time, and the bladder is often in a high-pressure state, which increases the burden on the bladder. In severe cases, it can affect the upper urinary tract, and CIC does not play a positive role; too frequent catheterizations, although the bladder pressure is reduced, may increase the probability of urethral injury and increase the inconvenience of the patient and parents. The appropriate frequency of catheterization is important for the successful implementation of CIC [9].

Parents of patients should be required to assist in recording a catheterization diary, guiding them on how to accurately record various data, such as water intake (including intake of various liquids and number of intakes), time and interval of each catheterization, volume of each catheterization, whether there is leakage, etc. The patient should drink water evenly to maintain a certain urine volume to prevent UTI and can adjust the water intake reasonably according to the urine volume, avoid taking a large amount of liquid in a short time, and try not to take liquid after dinner to prevent a large amount of urine from being produced at night. Although doctors often make strict drinking plans for patients in clinical practice, it is difficult to fully implement them in actual procedures, especially for infants and young children. Due to their own crying and other reasons, parents often disrupt the drinking plan. In addition, the production of urine is not only related to the amount of water intake but also to body position. Research by Shen Haitao and others suggests that patients produce more urine when lying flat than when sitting, and the time for urine production is shortened. In addition to implementing a water intake plan, it is also necessary to accurately measure the maximum bladder capacity and PVR of the children before catheterization.

When the pressure in the bladder exceeds 40 cmH_2O, the risk of upper urinary tract damage such as hydronephrosis increases [10]. 40 cmH_2O is the upper limit of safe bladder pressure. Safe bladder capacity (SBC) refers to the bladder capacity when the bladder filling pressure is below 40 cmH_2O. Storing and urinating under safe bladder pressure or not exceeding SBC can protect the upper urinary tract. Research suggests that a bladder capacity meter can be used for NB patients to timely measure the volume of urine in the bladder, which can guide the interval of CIC. This device, equivalent to a portable ultrasound, can allow the patients to catheterize before reaching SBC and achieve good results. However, this device requires assistance from parents or caregivers for measurement, and the patients cannot complete it themselves. These indicators can basically understand the function of the bladder and provide a basis for determining the interval of catheterization. For patients and their parents, mastering the interval of catheterization is a gradual training process. After a period of training, patients and their parents can generally master their own catheterization routine. The number of catheterizations is generally four to eight times a day, once after getting up in the morning and before going to bed at night and the rest of the time according to their own situation. For school-age children, they can catheterize during breaks. When the bladder is overly filled, the bladder mucosal folds decrease or disappear; the bladder wall vessels become thinner, finer, and longer; and the bladder storage pressure and abdominal pressure significantly increase. At this time, if the amount of urine catheterized at one time is too much, the bladder pressure drops sharply, which may damage the bladder mucosa and cause hematuria. Regular ultrasound and urodynamic study to measure the patient's maximum bladder capacity, SBC, and PVR changes can be performed once a year to check the upper urinary tract situation. According to these parameters, adjust the catheterization interval. If the single catheterization volume exceeds SBC, it will easily cause upper urinary tract damage such as hydronephrosis over time, and the catheterization interval needs to be shortened. Catheterize before the bladder is filled to a safe capacity to keep the bladder in a low-pressure state. Research by Wang Junxia and others shows that CIC combined with catheterization during sleep at night, compared with simple daytime CIC, SBC, and BC, will significantly increase, while the incidence of UTI did not significantly increase; VUR and hydronephrosis will also significantly improve, which helps to protect the upper urinary tract [11].

6.4 CIC Compliance of Children [12]

The premise of successful CIC is that the patient follows the doctor's instructions and cooperates with the doctor's treatment. For children, especially infants and young children, the coprocedure of parents is crucial. Only when the parents' compliance is high, the child's compliance be improved. If you want to improve the child's compliance, you must first improve the child and parents' understanding of the awareness of CIC, and doctors need to explain in detail the purpose and significance of CIC and guide patients on how to operate CIC and its long-term use.

The health-care worker guiding CIC can come from urology, rehabilitation departments, etc., but they must have daily catheterization experience and have undergone formal training.

Older children may think that CIC has increased their "patient role," affecting their compliance. Giving them more time will make it easier to accept CIC, and they can master this skill and improve the compliance of CIC. Children perform CIC at school, because the way of voiding is different from other classmates, need a separate enclosed public toilet, which may cause embarrassment, even shame, affecting the child's confidence. Children and parents may be afraid of repeatedly inserting the catheter into the urethra, causing UTI, pain, or irreversible damage to the urinary tract. The nerves in the urethra are indeed abundant, with sympathetic and parasympathetic nerves distributed throughout the urethra. The nerve distribution in the bladder neck is also abundant. The mucosa is very sensitive to stimuli. Foreign bodies or inflammatory reactions can stimulate and cause urinary pain, even causing discomfort in the perineum and lower abdomen. All of these can affect the quality of learning CIC. We need to make children and parents confident in the safety of CIC, inform them of precautions, and give encouragement. It is necessary to fully mobilize the enthusiasm of the parents of the patients, because children are young and their cognition and behavior abilities are not mature yet; they need the active participation and coprocedure of their parents, maintain patience, and give enough time to ensure the normal progress of CIC.

There are many factors affecting the compliance of children with CIC. Internal factors (related to the child) include physical obstacles, urethral orifice positioning obstacles, lack of flexibility, visual impairments (such as weak vision), anatomical abnormalities, psychological obstacles, intellectual disabilities or mental abnormalities, misunderstandings and anxiety, embarrassment and lack of confidence, shame, fear and pain, etc. External factors include caregiver factors, lack of enthusiasm, lack of time and patience, worry that the child cannot tolerate, low cognitive and behavioral abilities, instructor factors, inadequate training quality, lack of supervision and follow-up, social and economic factors, lack of independent enclosed public toilets, high cost of catheter use, etc.

The inability to find a suitable and correct catheter is also a reason why CIC cannot be performed. The size, type, and material of the catheter affect the comfort of the child. It is crucial to choose a catheter that can be used comfortably. Using a hydrophilic-coated catheter can provide more comfort and ease of use. Many catheters used for CIC are disposable, and there are various types of catheters available, each with its own characteristics. The price of the catheter should be considered, and the parents of the patient can choose a catheter that their financial situation can afford. Health-care workers can recommend the catheter they think is most suitable based on their experience. The choice of catheter for infants and young children should be particularly careful, and as small a catheter as possible should be chosen to protect the child's urethra, prevent injury, and increase the confidence of the parents to improve compliance. Lack of proper training is also a major obstacle to the success of CIC. For infant and young child patients, their parents should be trained. For older children, both parents and children should receive training. Some people may only need one training session to learn, while others may need multiple training sessions to master. This requires experienced trainers to spend enough time communicating with patients, introducing them to various types of catheters, and demonstrating catheterization procedures. The training environment should be quiet and private, protecting patient privacy and dignity. Continuous professional support and advice are crucial for patients compliance. Initially, the procedure should be supervised by the instructor, correcting any incorrect procedures in a timely manner. Later, regular follow-ups should be made to monitor the child's use of CIC and any problems encountered, to ensure that the child is always using the correct procedure technique, and to understand changes in the child's voiding function, record the child's catheterization diary, and regularly conduct various urinary system examinations to provide guidance and advice for adjusting the child's catheterization plan.

6.5 Complications of CIC in Children [13]

Long-term use of CIC in children is relatively safe, and complications are rare. Long-term follow-up studies at home and abroad show that the education of professional treatment and nursing staff to CIC patients and their families is crucial for the protection of the child's bladder and kidney function. Faure and others studied 60 male CIC patients. Long-term follow-up (8.2 ± 1.4 years) studies found that CIC is effective and safe in protecting the kidney and bladder function of patients, and with the education of health-care worker, the compliance of patients is good.

6.5.1 Urinary Tract Infection [14]

UTI is the most common complication in children with CIC. If the urine has a foul smell and is obviously turbid and there is recurrent fever, urethral pain, perineal discomfort, lower abdominal pain, or back pain during catheterization, it may indicate the occurrence of UTI. Mild cases can be relieved by drinking more water and shortening the catheterization interval, while severe cases require oral or intravenous antibiotics to control the infection, and a catheter may need to be left in place until symptoms disappear. Although CIC may have some complications such as UTI, it is safer and more reliable compared to indwelling catheters.

Because bacteria can enter the bladder through the inner lumen (inner surface of the catheter) or the outer layer of the catheter during the insertion process, bacteriuria may form, but it is easy to treat. With regular and timely catheterization, the bacteria in the bladder will continuously decrease and dilute, not enough to cause an infection that damages the bladder mucosa. Asymptomatic bacteriuria is more common, while those with high fever or pyelonephritis are rare and do not have serious consequences for CIC treatment.

A low frequency of catheterization and long intervals can lead to over-expansion of the bladder, and long-term urinary retention can increase the risk of UTIs. Therefore, the child and caregiver can keep a catheterization diary, regularly empty the bladder as planned, and reduce the risk of UTIs caused by urinary retention and bacteriuria. If the child drinks too little water, the production of urine will decrease, which will reduce the frequency of voiding, prolong the residual time of urine in the bladder, or not completely empty the bladder during catheterization, which can easily provide a suitable environment for bacterial growth. Therefore, it is necessary to drink water evenly and appropriately, but avoid excessive drinking, avoid liquid intake after dinner, and be patient during catheterization to ensure full bladder drainage. Non-standard CIC techniques can contaminate the catheter and mistakenly introduce bacteria into the bladder, causing UTIs. Therefore, it is necessary to standardize the training of catheterization techniques, thoroughly wash hands before starting catheterization, thoroughly clean the genital area and perineal area with soap and water every day, avoid touching the tip of the catheter, avoid letting the catheter touch other surfaces, and use lubricant for children who have difficulty inserting the catheter. Low immunity or other underlying diseases may increase the risk of UTIs, so it is necessary to improve physical fitness and immunity. The child needs to regularly undergo urinary routine, urine culture, and other urinary system examinations to detect and treat early, reducing the damage of complications.

6.5.2 Urethral Injury

The child's urethra is more delicate than an adult's, and repeated catheterization can potentially injure the child's urethra, leading to urethral stricture and the formation of false urethral passage. This is not easy to occur in the short term, but the incidence will increase with the extension of CIC time. If blood is found in the catheter or urine during catheterization, a small amount may be due to urethral mucosal injury. If there is a large amount of bleeding or continuous bleeding, catheterization should be stopped immediately, and medical attention should be sought. Using a hydrophilic-coated catheter or a regular catheter that is fully lubricated can reduce the risk of urethral stricture or false passage injuries, and the catheterization action should be gentle. If a urethral fistula occurs, antibiotics can be used for treatment, and a catheter should be left in place for drainage until the urethral fistula is healed before continuing with CIC.

6.5.3 Psychological Disorders

After a long period of CIC, the child may develop psychological disorders such as inferiority, autism, anxiety, and depression due to the different voiding methods compared to other children of the same age, which may due to a closed environment for voiding. As a result, they become more isolated and less sociable, and it even affects their academic performance. Therefore, for these children, it is necessary to regularly assess their psychological state, actively guide them to integrate into their surrounding living and learning environment, and parents should communicate with the school teachers about the actual situation of the child. When the parents are not around, the teacher is responsible for supervising and managing the child's catheterization and psychological condition.

6.6 Promotion and Education of Children's CIC

Due to the need for long-term continuous treatment, the health-care worker guiding the child must possess the corresponding abilities, necessary knowledge, and a good attitude to maintain treatment and adapt to changes in the environment of the child and their parents. As children's CIC is often operated by the child's parents or the child themselves, compliance is poor; therefore, good propaganda and education are particularly important. Detailed patient information is also important for the successful implementation of CIC. Doctors should first assess the child's condition and the parents' understanding of the disease and urinary anatomy, inform the child and parents of the necessity and importance of CIC, then inform them of the detailed procedure methods and procedures, recommend suitable catheters according to the family's economic conditions, pay attention to the method, promote an environment that protects the child's privacy, and create a relaxed atmosphere. Through various forms and rich content of health education, the child's compliance can be improved; relevant promotional materials, lower urinary tract anatomy diagrams, anatomical models, and other visual aids can be provided to the child and parents, and it is best to show them instructional videos for intuitive learning; instructional videos are very helpful for children learning CIC, but they cannot replace face-to-face communication and learning with doctors. The application of technologies such as instructional videos allows professionals to share knowledge, promote discussion, and encourage participation from the child and parents. Through these means, the child can master the correct procedure methods, encourage the good aspects, analyze and correct the problems that arise, and build confidence in the child and parents. Some children cannot correctly understand their disease because they do not accept CIC internally, so it is necessary to educate the child psychologically, strive to get the support of the parents, and involve the parents, and with the coprocedure of the parents, the child can change from passively accepting CIC to actively and positively carrying it out. Successful cases can be introduced to them, patient groups can be established, communication between the child and their parents can be promoted, and their tension, fear, and anxiety can be eliminated. At the same time, the child should be instructed to improve their physical fitness, strengthen nutrition, and increase immunity. During the process of CIC, doctors should also advise the child and parents on how to prevent and detect UTI and other potential complications, when to undergo urinary system examinations, how to collect urine samples, and when necessary to obtain treatment. Currently, the procedure and specific requirements of CIC lack unified standards and guidelines; relevant health education materials, especially instructional videos, are relatively scarce, and further development is needed; relevant patient communication platforms are also few, and more improvements are needed.

In conclusion, CIC is currently the preferred method of bladder emptying recommended by ICS and is increasingly used in clinical practice. For children with NB, early diagnosis, early treatment, and early initiation of CIC are essential. Therefore, it is necessary to carry out CIC publicity and education work; formulate individualized education plans according to the patient's age, personality, and parents' level of education; determine the catheterization interval time according to the child's own situation; cooperate with the drinking water plan; record the catheterization diary; adhere to the correct CIC method and process; choose the appropriate catheter; and reduce the occurrence of the risk of various complications; regular telephone or face-to-face follow-up, communication of problems encountered in the child's catheterization and resolution, regular urinalysis, urine culture, urinary system ultrasound, urodynamics and other urinary system examinations, and timely adjustment of CIC plan according to the changes in the condition are important. CIC helps to stabilize the upper urinary tract, can reduce the child's dependence on health-care workers, can improve the child's independence, is conducive to the child's return to the family and integration into society, and truly improves the child's quality of life. However, how to improve the child's adherence to CIC is still worth further exploration, and more prospective studies on the long-term efficacy and complications of CIC in children with NB are needed in the future to provide a basis for the rational application of CIC.

Date	Time	CIC Urine Volume (mL)	Amount of Urine leakage on Diaper or Pants (None; Small; Medium; Large)

Fig. 6.14 CIC recording form in children

Table 6.1 Basic skills and knowledge of CIC

1. How to properly clean hands
2. Master the types and sizes of catheters
3. How to lubricate the catheter and insert it into the urethra
4. How to measure the amount of each catheterization
5. How to identify symptoms of urinary tract infection in children
6. Understanding when to seek medical attention

6.7 Common Tables for Children's CIC

This section introduces some commonly used tables to guide children and parents in CIC, to facilitate parents' care for their children.

Parents need to record the daily CIC situation for children, which is beneficial for doctors to understand the child's daily CIC situation and can provide targeted guidance for the children's renal function and bladder function through the amount of each CIC catheterization. The specific recording method can be seen in Fig. 6.14. Parents of the child should master common CIC knowledge to ensure that they can handle common CIC problems correctly, as detailed in Table 6.1.

References

1. Prieto JA, Murphy CL, Stewart F, Fader M. Intermittent catheter techniques, strategies and designs for managing long-term bladder conditions [J]. Cochrane Database Syst Rev. 2021;10(10):CD006008.
2. Guerra L, Leonard M, Castagnetti M. Best practice in the assessment of bladder function in infants [J]. Ther Adv Urol. 2014;6(4):148–64. https://doi.org/10.1177/1756287214528745.
3. Maison POM, Lazarus J. The management of paediatric neurogenic bladder: an approach in a resource-poor setting [J]. Paediatr Int Child Health. 2017;37(4):280–5. https://doi.org/10.1080/20469047.2017.1351745.
4. Kim JK, Khondker A, Chua ME, et al. Assessing the utility of tamsulosin in delaying progression to clean intermittent catheterization and end-stage renal disease in patients with posterior urethral valves: are we postponing the inevitable? [J]. Urology. 2023;179:151–7.
5. Lamin E, Newman DK. Clean intermittent catheterization revisited [J]. Int Urol Nephrol. 2016;48(6):931–9. https://doi.org/10.1007/s11255-016-1236-9.
6. De Castro R, Fouda Neel KA, Alshammari AM, et al. Clean intermittent catheterization in Saudi children. Suggestion for a common protocol [J]. Saudi Med J. 2000;21(11):1016–23.
7. Aslan AR, Kogan BA. Conservative management in neurogenic bladder dysfunction [J]. Curr Opin Urol. 2002;12(6):473–7. https://doi.org/10.1097/00042307-200211000-00005.
8. Segal ES, Deatrick JA, Hagelgans NA. The determinants of successful self-catheterization programs in children with myelomeningoceles [J]. J Pediatr Nurs. 1995;10(2):82–8. https://doi.org/10.1016/s0882-5963(05)80002-8.
9. Jeong SJ, Oh SJ. Recent updates in urinary catheter products for the neurogenic bladder patients with spinal cord injury [J]. Korean J Neurotrauma. 2019;15(2):77–87. https://doi.org/10.13004/kjnt.2019.15.e41.
10. Tenke P, Köves B, Johansen TE. An update on prevention and treatment of catheter-associated urinary tract infections [J]. Curr Opin Infect Dis. 2014;27(1):102–7. https://doi.org/10.1097/qco.0000000000000031.

11. Chenoweth CE, Saint S. Urinary tract infections [J]. Infect Dis Clin N Am. 2011;25(1):103–15. https://doi.org/10.1016/j.idc.2010.11.005.
12. Li Y, Stern N, Wang PZ, et al. Systematic review and meta-analysis to study the outcomes of proactive versus delayed management in children with a congenital neurogenic bladder [J]. J Pediatr Urol. 2023;19(6):730–41. https://doi.org/10.1016/j.jpurol.2023.08.033.
13. Lucas E. Medical management of neurogenic bladder for children and adults: a review [J]. Top Spinal Cord Inj Rehabil. 2019;25(3):195–204. https://doi.org/10.1310/sci2503-195.
14. Saadat SH, Shepherd S, Van Asseldonk B, Elterman DS. Clean intermittent catheterization: single use vs. reuse [J]. Can Urol Assoc J. 2019;13(2):64–9.

7 Partial (Morning and Evening) CIC for Patients with Partial Bladder Emptying Disorders

Jian-Guo Wen

CIC is often used for patients with NB who cannot excrete enough urine [1]. By regularly inserting a disposable catheter into the urethra or bladder diversion four to six times a day to empty the urine, the bladder capacity is controlled within a safe capacity, and the bladder pressure is controlled within a safe pressure range, to avoid complications such as upper urinary tract dilation [2], ureteral reflux [3], hydronephrosis [4], and renal failure [2] caused by long-term high bladder pressure. Internationally, the use of CIC is recommended. As the preferred treatment method for patients who cannot fully and safely empty their bladder, especially for those with neurogenic voiding dysfunction, it is an effective measure to achieve urinary bladder control [5]. According to literature, the indications for CIC are very broad [6], but for patients who have not completely lost bladder voiding function, they can use partial or only morning and evening CIC (also called morning and evening CIC). These methods that do not have to rely entirely on CIC for urination are called partial CIC or timed CIC (selected time clean intermittent catheterization, STCIC) or morning and evening CIC (morning evening CIC, MECIC), or morning, noon, and evening CIC (morning evening noon CIC, MENCIC). The purpose of STCIC is to prevent and treat a series of complications caused by excessive PVR leading to high bladder pressure (enuresis, urinary incontinence, etc.), protect the kidneys, and improve the quality of life. With a limited number of catheterizations per day (two to three times), it can control abnormal voiding symptoms and reduce catheter-induced UTI.

7.1 STCIC Indications

The choice of STCIC depends on the patient's symptoms, the degree of urinary function impairment, UDC results, and whether the patient cooperates, and the decisive factors include whether there is still a certain ability to urinate [7], the amount of PVR [8], whether there is urinary incontinence [9], urinary tract infection [10], upper urinary tract dilation [11], etc. PVR greater than 1/3 of the maximum bladder capacity or adult bladder PVR greater than 150 mL and recurrent UTI, enuresis, and/or nocturnal polyuria, daytime urinary incontinence, etc. and ineffective drug treatment are all indications for STCIC. STCIC can effectively reduce bladder pressure, so urodynamic tests showing high bladder pressure (bladder filling end detrusor pressure > 30 cmH_2O) [12] should also consider using STCIC. STCIC can effectively relieve high pressure in the bladder, avoid long-term high pressure in the bladder and progressive fibrosis of

J.-G. Wen (✉)
Pediatric Urodynamic Center/Department of Urology, First Affiliated Hospital of Zhengzhou University, Zhengzhou, China

J.-G. Wen (ed.), *Progress in Clean Intermittent Catheterization*, Experts' Perspectives on Medical Advances, https://doi.org/10.1007/978-981-97-5021-4_7

the bladder [13], and prevent VUR, upper urinary tract dilation or hydronephrosis, and other complications. Patients with stress incontinence can choose to empty the bladder at regular intervals every day to increase the functional bladder capacity, avoid overflow incontinence, reduce the occurrence of bladder damage and other complications in patients, and improve the quality of life of patients.

The key to STCIC is to use the catheter flexibly to keep the bladder capacity within the principle of safe capacity to empty the bladder, thereby effectively protecting the patient's bladder and upper urinary tract function at the same time. To maximize the quality of life of patients, reduce the risk of infection caused by complete reliance on CIC or long-term indwelling catheter, and avoid the embarrassment of patients carrying urine bags with them; it plays a transitional or alternative treatment role for patients' diseases.

7.1.1 Increased PVR

An increased PVR refers to the remaining urine in the bladder after natural voiding, indicating that the bladder has not completely emptied [14]. Normally, people can completely empty their bladder, making the PVR zero [15]. Normal newborns and infants may occasionally have an increased PVR [16]. Therefore, to clinically determine whether they have an increased PVR, at least two measurements of PVR are needed. As age increases and bladder function declines in the elderly, the PVR will correspondingly increase, but it generally should not exceed 20 mL. Otherwise, it suggests the presence of a pathological condition. Increased PVR is common in detrusor dysfunction [17], BOO [18], and postoperative conditions [19]. Long-term increase in bladder PVR, with urine accumulating in the bladder unable to be expelled, can lead to urinary tract infections, bladder stones, etc. Long-term high pressure in the bladder can also lead to upper urinary tract dilation, VUR, and even hydronephrosis and may cause a series of lower urinary tract symptoms such as urinary retention, enuresis, urgency, frequency, and incontinence, as well as abdominal distension, lower abdominal discomfort, and other symptoms. Common causes of increased PVR are as follows:

1. Detrusor dysfunction: such as weak detrusor or low tension of the detrusor, which means the bladder does not have enough power and endurance to empty the urine. This is often seen in neurogenic disorders or congenital diseases, such as stroke, Parkinson's syndrome [20], multiple sclerosis [21], diabetes [22], spinal cord lesions caused by trauma [23] or other diseases, and spinal cord meningocele [24] as well as posterior urethral valve in children [25], etc.
2. BOO: Even though the function of the detrusor is normal or only slightly weakened, the obstruction at the bladder outlet can still cause an increase in PVR. This is often seen in conditions like prostate hyperplasia, elevated bladder neck in women, urethral stricture, and urethral valve [26]. Male urethral stricture is often due to benign prostatic hyperplasia, as well as persistent infection and physiological structural changes caused by transurethral resection of the prostate or radical prostatectomy. Women may have congenital anatomical abnormalities such as a high bladder neck that cause incomplete bladder emptying. Since the vagina and urethra are adjacent in women, some women may develop structural abnormalities such as urethral bending due to uterine prolapse after childbirth, which can lead to voiding dysfunction.
3. Detrusor-sphincter dyssynergia: This refers to the involuntary contraction of the external urethral sphincter when the detrusor contracts. It can cause voiding dysfunction and can lead to reflux nephropathy and renal failure. It is often seen in patients with spinal cord injuries. Previous antispasmodic drug treatments were often unsatisfactory, but combining with CIC can reduce the occurrence of complications.
4. Postoperative voiding dysfunction: Any surgery to treat urinary incontinence carries the risk of bladder emptying disorders, and acute

urinary retention is also common after surgery, especially in surgeries using epidural anesthesia [27]. Surgeries to treat stress urinary incontinence, such as various sling surgeries, vaginal suspension surgeries, and fascial suspension surgeries, all carry the risk of postoperative urinary retention. Therefore, preoperative urodynamic testing of detrusor function can effectively assess the occurrence of voiding dysfunction after incontinence surgery. Other surgeries include bladder reconstruction, diversion, etc. A bladder or bladder substitute with a valve can be closed normally and opened and inserted with a catheter when needed for CIC, thus achieving urine discharge.

7.1.2 Overflow Incontinence

Overflow incontinence refers to chronic urinary retention caused by urethral obstruction (urethral stricture, bladder neck spasm, and prostate hyperplasia, etc.) and bladder underactivity [28]. When the bladder is overly filled, the pressure inside the bladder exceeds the resistance of the normal urethral sphincter, and urine uncontrollably overflows from the urethra. Clinically, it manifests as incontinence, increased nocturia, and nocturnal enuresis. Long-term elevated bladder pressure can cause upper urinary tract obstruction and damage kidney function. Common clinical causes include prostate hyperplasia and NB. Overflow incontinence is prone to urinary tract infections and stones due to the bladder being in a filled state (increased PVR) for a long time.

There are many causes of overflow incontinence [29], such as urinary retention caused by NB, prostate hyperplasia, or bladder neck spasm or urethral stricture, unstable bladder, weakened sphincter function due to weakened pelvic floor muscle tension in postmenopausal women or uterine prolapse and bladder protrusion after childbirth, various pelvic surgeries, etc. [30]. This type of incontinence can use CIC in conjunction with a drinking plan to achieve regular bladder emptying, thereby relieving the patient's embarrassing situation of incontinence. If the patient still has partial voiding function, STCIC treatment can be considered when the effect of drug or surgical treatment is not satisfactory. The common method is to catheterize three times a day, i.e., before going to bed at night, after getting up in the morning, and before noon break for CIC, and encourage self-voiding and multiple voiding at other times.

7.2 STCIC Precautions

1. The frequency of STCIC is determined by the degree of voiding dysfunction, the impact on quality of life, frequency-volume chart, bladder functional capacity, ultrasound scan PVR, and other comprehensive assessments. The principle is to avoid bladder capacity exceeding 400–500 mL. When the urine to be drained less than 100 mL or more than 500 mL, it should be considered to adjust the frequency and interval of catheterization or water intake, and formulate the least and most convenient catheterization plan every day.
2. UDS can provide guidance. Through UDS, the patient's detrusor function, bladder capacity, reflux, type of urinary incontinence, etc. can be assessed.
3. Keeping a voiding diary and regularly visiting the outpatient clinic are the key to timely adjustment of the catheterization plan to ensure the safety of the patient's bladder. Long-term persistence and vigilance are the keys to successful use of CIC.
4. The key to STCIC is to flexibly formulate a timed voiding plan after a detailed assessment, which needs to be flexibly used under the guidance of a professional urologist to assist in the treatment and recovery of the disease.

7.3 Timed CIC Cases

Case 1: Male, 60 years old, visited the outpatient clinic with "frequent voiding, urgency, incomplete voiding for 3 years, accompanied by lower abdominal discomfort and nocturnal enuresis for 2 days." Abdominal ultrasound, prostate digital examination, and routine urine and prostate fluid tests suggested prostate hyperplasia, urinary system infection, PVR of about 200 mL, mild hydronephrosis in the right kidney, and prostatitis. Previously, oral medication for treating prostate hyperplasia was ineffective. The patient can urinate on his own, but 2 days ago, the patient suddenly had a decrease in urine volume and dysuria.

Treatment suggestion: After controlling the infection, surgical treatment is needed to relieve the obstruction. Considering the patient refused to keep the catheter, so it was suggested to perform CIC at a fixed time every day, once in the morning and once before going to bed at night, control water intake and drug treatment, and reassess whether surgery can be performed after 2 weeks.

Case 2: Male, 58 years old, due to a car accident caused "T10 vertebral body comminuted fracture with complete dislocation," underwent "T10 vertebral fracture with dislocation reduction + internal fixation surgery" 2 months ago. Now he can sit for several hours with the support of a thoracolumbar brace and both hands, but he cannot stand or walk; he can partially urinate, but the urine volume is small. Abdominal ultrasound showed: "Increased PVR in the bladder is about 210 mL, no VUR, no kidney damage." UDS indicated that the detrusor did not contract, the bladder was filled to 500 mL, the detrusor pressure rose to 40 cmH_2O, and overflow incontinence occurred. He can void with abdominal pressure, but there is a lot of PVR after voiding, which is confirmed by ultrasound.

Treatment suggestion: Perform CIC at a fixed time every day, once in the morning and once before going to bed at night. At other times, encourage the patient to urinate with abdominal pressure. Keep a voiding diary to understand the pattern of drinking water and voiding, and find a reasonable interval for abdominal pressure voiding under the safe bladder capacity. There should be regular follow-up and urinary system ultrasound examination.

Case 3: Female, aged 8, sought treatment for "nocturnal enuresis (NE) since childhood." The child has no urinary incontinence during the day. She reported being able to urinate on her own. After birth, the child had surgery for congenital spinal meningocele. There was no significant improvement after 2 months of medication for enuresis. Ultrasound examination showed that the bladder wall was not smooth, with PVR of 100 mL, and no obvious abnormalities in the kidneys.

Diagnosis and treatment suggestions: The child has a NB caused by spina bifida, so the suggested diagnosis and treatment measures are (1) VUDS to assess the condition of the detrusor and sphincter, bladder compliance, and whether there is VUR, etc.; (2) prohibit holding urine and encourage frequent voiding, such as going to the toilet during breaks and urinating within 1 hour after meals; (3) perform CIC regularly every day, once in the morning and once before going to bed; (4) adjust the treatment plan according to the results of the UDS; (5) routine urine tests to rule out UTI; (6) keep a voiding (catheterization) diary to guide CIC.

7.4 Summary

In summary, STCIC is a part of CIC, mainly suitable for patients who can still urinate on their own (or abdominal pressure voiding) but have significantly increased PVR, especially accompanied by urinary incontinence and recurrent UTI history and ineffective drug treatment. STCIC mainly refers to performing CIC once before going to bed at night and once when getting up in the morning. Use a limited number of catheterizations to treat significant increases in PVR and the resulting overflow incontinence and urinary system infections, prevent damage to the upper urinary tract, and create conditions for the recovery of bladder function.

References

1. Rehabilitation Nursing Professional Committee, Chinese Association of Rehabilitation Medicine. Neurogenic bladder care practice guidelines (2017 edition) [J]. J Nurs Sci. 2017;32(24):1–7. https://doi.org/10.3870/j.issn.1001-4152.2017.24.001. [

中国康复医学会康复护理专业委员会. 神经源性膀胱护理实践指南(2017年版). 护理学杂志, 2017;32(24):1–7].
2. Amarenco G, Sheikh Ismaël S, Chesnel C, et al. Diagnosis and clinical evaluation of neurogenic bladder [J]. Eur J Phys Rehabil Med. 2017;53(6):975–80. https://doi.org/10.23736/s1973-9087.17.04992-9.
3. Acar B, Arikan FI, Germiyanoğlu C, Dallar Y. Influence of high bladder pressure on vesicoureteral reflux and its resolution [J]. Urol Int. 2009;82(1):77–80. https://doi.org/10.1159/000176030.
4. Huen KH, Chamberlin JD, Macaraeg A, et al. Home bladder pressure measurements correlate with urodynamic storage pressures and high-grade hydronephrosis in children with spina bifida [J]. J Pediatr Urol. 2022;18(4):503.e501–7. https://doi.org/10.1016/j.jpurol.2022.06.011.
5. Vahr S, Cobussen-Boekhorst H, Eikenboom J, et al. Catheterisation: urethral intermittent in adults. Dilatation, urethral intermittent in adults. EAUN guideline. EAUN; 2013.
6. Di Benedetto P. Clean intermittent self-catheterization in neuro-urology [J]. Eur J Phys Rehabil Med. 2011;47(4):651–9.
7. Roshanzamir F, Rouzrokh M, Mirshemirani A, et al. Treatment outcome of neurogenic bladder dysfunction in children; a five-year experience [J]. Iran J Pediatr. 2014;24(3):323–6.
8. Wang QW, Wen JG, Song DK, et al. Is it possible to use urodynamic variables to predict upper urinary tract dilatation in children with neurogenic bladder-sphincter dysfunction? [J]. BJU Int. 2006;98(6):1295–300. https://doi.org/10.1111/j.1464-410X.2006.06402.x.
9. Kennelly M, Cruz F, Herschorn S, et al. Efficacy and safety of abobotulinumtoxinA in patients with neurogenic detrusor overactivity incontinence performing regular clean intermittent catheterization: pooled results from two phase 3 randomized studies (CONTENT1 and CONTENT2) [J]. Eur Urol. 2022;82(2):223–32. https://doi.org/10.1016/j.eururo.2022.03.010.
10. Edokpolo LU, Stavris KB, Foster HE Jr. Intermittent catheterization and recurrent urinary tract infection in spinal cord injury [J]. Top Spinal Cord Inj Rehabil. 2012;18(2):187–92. https://doi.org/10.1310/sci1802-187.
11. Obara K, Komeyama T, Mizusawa T, et al. [The consequence after introduction of clean intermittent catheterization (CIC) in children with neurogenic bladder dysfunction secondary to spina bifida--the comparison of patients with and without upper urinary tract dilation at the time CIC was introduced] [J]. Nihon Hinyokika Gakkai Zasshi. 2003;94(7):664–70. https://doi.org/10.5980/jpnjurol1989.94.664.
12. Hogg FRA, Kearney S, Solomon E, et al. Acute, severe traumatic spinal cord injury: improving urinary bladder function by optimizing spinal cord perfusion [J]. J Neurosurg Spine. 2022;36(1):145–52. https://doi.org/10.3171/2021.3.Spine202056.
13. Elzeneini W, Waly R, Marshall D, Bailie A. Early start of clean intermittent catheterization versus expectant management in children with spina bifida [J]. J Pediatr Surg. 2019;54(2):322–5. https://doi.org/10.1016/j.jpedsurg.2018.10.096.
14. Li Q, Wen Y, Zhang R, et al. Analysis of urine flow rate and post-voiding residual urine volume results under first desire to void versus strong desire to void [J]. J Clin Pediatr Surg. 2018;17(7):492–5. https://doi.org/10.3969/j.issn.1671-6353.2018.07.004. [李琦,文一博,张瑞莉,等. 遗尿患儿初始尿意与强烈尿意时尿流率及残余尿测定分析. 临床小儿外科杂志, 2018;17(7):492–5].
15. Uzun H, Kadioglu ME, Metin NO, Akca G. The association of postvoiding residual volume, uroflowmetry parameters and bladder sensation [J]. Urol J. 2019;16(4):403–6. https://doi.org/10.22037/uj.v0i0.4368.
16. Van Der Cruyssen K, De Wachter S, Van Hal G, et al. The voiding pattern in healthy pre- and term infants and toddlers: a literature review [J]. Eur J Pediatr. 2015;174(9):1129–42. https://doi.org/10.1007/s00431-015-2578-5.
17. Kaplan SA, Wein AJ, Staskin DR, et al. Urinary retention and post-void residual urine in men: separating truth from tradition [J]. J Urol. 2008;180(1):47–54. https://doi.org/10.1016/j.juro.2008.03.027.
18. Verhovsky G, Baberashvili I, Rappaport YH, et al. Bladder oversensitivity is associated with bladder outlet obstruction in men [J]. J Pers Med. 2022;12(10):1675. https://doi.org/10.3390/jpm12101675.
19. Toyama Y, Suzuki Y, Nakayama S, et al. Outcome of modified laparoscopic sacrocolpopexy and its effect on voiding dysfunction [J]. J Nippon Med Sch. 2022;89(2):222–6. https://doi.org/10.1272/jnms.JNMS.2022_89-219.
20. Hu JC, Hsu LN, Lee WC, et al. Role of urological botulinum toxin-A injection for overactive bladder and voiding dysfunction in patients with Parkinson's disease or post-stroke [J]. Toxins (Basel). 2023;15(2):166. https://doi.org/10.3390/toxins15020166.
21. Vecchio M, Chiaramonte R, Benedetto PDI. Management of bladder dysfunction in multiple sclerosis: a systematic review and meta-analysis of studies regarding bladder rehabilitation [J]. Eur J Phys Rehabil Med. 2022;58(3):387–96. https://doi.org/10.23736/s1973-9087.22.07217-3.
22. Liu G, Daneshgari F. Diabetic bladder dysfunction [J]. Chin Med J. 2014;127(7):1357–64.
23. Cruz CD, Coelho A, Antunes-Lopes T, Cruz F. Biomarkers of spinal cord injury and ensuing bladder dysfunction [J]. Adv Drug Deliv Rev. 2015;82–83:153–9. https://doi.org/10.1016/j.addr.2014.11.007.
24. Rendeli C, Ausili E, Tabacco F, et al. Urodynamic evaluation in children with lipomeningocele: timing for neurosurgery, spinal cord tethering and followup [J]. J Urol. 2007;177(6):2319–24. https://doi.org/10.1016/j.juro.2007.01.176.

25. Taskinen S, Heikkilä J, Rintala R. Posterior urethral valves: primary voiding pressures and kidney function in infants [J]. J Urol. 2009;182(2):699–702; discussion 702–3. https://doi.org/10.1016/j.juro.2009.04.035.
26. Mardy A. Bladder outlet obstruction [J]. Am J Obstet Gynecol. 2021;225(5):B9–B11. https://doi.org/10.1016/j.ajog.2021.06.039.
27. Yeung JH, Gates S, Naidu BV, et al. Paravertebral block versus thoracic epidural for patients undergoing thoracotomy [J]. Cochrane Database Syst Rev. 2016;2(2):CD009121. https://doi.org/10.1002/14651858.CD009121.pub2.
28. Khandelwal C, Kistler C. Diagnosis of urinary incontinence [J]. Am Fam Physician. 2013;87(8):543–50.
29. Bardsley A. An overview of urinary incontinence [J]. Br J Nurs. 2016;25(18):S14–21. https://doi.org/10.12968/bjon.2016.25.18.S14.
30. Liu K, Wen J, Zhang P, et al. Urodynamic analysis in female patients with overflow incontinence complicated with upper urinary tract dilatation [J]. J Zhejiang Univ (Med Sci). 2006;41(2):212–4. https://doi.org/10.13705/j.issn.1671-6825.2006.02.006. [刘奎,文建国,张鹏,等. 女性充溢性尿失禁上尿路扩张患者尿动力学分析. 郑州大学学报(医学版), 2006;41(2):212–4].

8 CIC Combined with Urinary Diversion Effectively Improve the Bladder Control

Jian-Guo Wen

CIC is a common method for paralytic bladder patients to empty their bladder. There are clear procedures and guidelines for CIC performed through the urethra. However, for special cases such as patients with urinary diversion [1], there is still a need to strengthen guidance and training for CIC to empty the bladder. CIC combined with urinary diversion can effectively solve the urinary bladder control problem for these patients [2–4]. Here, we introduce the training and procedure key points for CIC after urinary diversion surgery.

8.1 Urinary Diversion Surgery

Urinary diversion surgery refers to the surgical method where urine needs to be discharged from a newly established channel due to various reasons [5]. Common ones include the following:

1. Mitrofanoff method (appendix cystostomy) [6]: a small tube (such as the appendix) is fixed between the mucosa and muscle layer of the bladder or urinary reservoir; if there is no appendix, fallopian tubes and ureters can be used, a certain length of ileum can be sewn into an appropriate diameter output channel, connecting the bladder and the abdominal wall.
2. Kock method [7]: the ileum is made into a stacked artificial valve.
3. Indiana method [8]: ileocecal valve is used for bladder enlargement and urinary diversion.

After bladder augmentation and controllable urinary diversion or simply controllable urinary diversion, CIC needs to be performed through the new bladder outlet.

Generally, for surgeries using the appendix as the urethra [9], catheterization is done from the navel. Although the catheterization method is different from the common urethral catheterization, it is more convenient. To perform catheterization through the umbilical appendix channel well, one must first understand the surgery using the appendix as the urethra. In cases of bladder eversion [10], NB [11], and bladder resection [12], bladder enlargement or reconstruction often uses the in situ appendix output channel controllable ileocecal colon bladder surgery, commonly using the appendix or ileum to create a stoma from the navel or upper abdomen [13]. Now, taking the Mitrofanoff method as an example, we introduce the surgical process to better understand the anatomy and function of the newly established bladder outlet.

Mitrofanoff procedure [14–17]: The surgery takes a midline incision in the lower abdomen, finds the appendix, and frees the appendix with

J.-G. Wen (✉)
Pediatric Urodynamic Center/Department of Urology, First Affiliated Hospital of Zhengzhou University, Zhengzhou, China

J.-G. Wen (ed.), *Progress in Clean Intermittent Catheterization*, Experts' Perspectives on Medical Advances, https://doi.org/10.1007/978-981-97-5021-4_8

3–4 cm of the cecal wall. If the appendix cannot be used, the ileum can be chosen, freeing 2.5 cm of the ileum, longitudinally cut and then transversely wrapped around a 16 Fr silicone tube, intermittently sutured with absorbable thread, forming a 7 cm long tube (Monti tube). One end of the Monti tube is implanted in the urinary reservoir, and the other end is fixed to the skin. The Monti tube is implanted in the submucosal layer of the new bladder, and a tunnel anastomosis is performed to control urinary incontinence. The new urinary reservoir can be made from the ileum or colon into a spherical new bladder. In this way, the new urethra is formed by the Monti tube made from the appendix or ileum; one end opens at the navel or a higher position, mainly for convenient catheterization; and one end opens under the mucosa of the new bladder, with a length of 7–10 cm, and the path is from the navel through the subcutaneous transverse rectus abdominis to the abdominal cavity and then to the submucosa of the bladder. At this time, urine can be stored in the new bladder or the original bladder but will not flow out from the new channel. When urinating, a catheter needs to be inserted into the new controllable channel to urinate. This is when CIC is needed.

In order to achieve controllable urinary diversion, it is generally necessary to perform a "VQZ" stoma surgery that can insert a catheter based on urinary diversion [18]. The "VQZ" (V-shaped-Quadrilateral-Z-shaped) stoma surgery is suitable for Mitrofanoff surgery or colostomy surgery that involves skin stomas. This type of stoma surgery has more advantages than direct skin stomas [19]. First, it is more concealed and does not attract people's attention; second, it does not expose the mucosa, thus protecting the mucosa; finally, the junction of the mucosa and skin is a very long suture area, and this suture area is not circular, thereby reducing the risk of stoma stenosis.

The method of making the "VQZ" stoma surgery mainly includes the following steps [20]: (1) Cut the skin and subcutaneous tissue to form a V-shaped flap. It is very important to determine the position of the flap, which should be at the bottom rather than the top of the planned stoma. The vertical axis of the V-shaped flap should form a smaller side angle with the projection line of the appendix on the body surface. (2) Lift the V-shaped flap, separate the abdominal wall muscles to form a larger gap, and pull the appendix out from it. (3) After the incision is closed, the appendix is pulled out of the incision and cut along its mesenteric edge. (4) Insert the V-shaped flap into the appendix hole and suture with 5-0 suture. (5) After the insertion of the V-shaped flap is completed, a quadrilateral flap is made from the upper edge of the abdominal wall defect of the V-shaped flap. If there are scars on the abdominal wall, an additional inside Z-shaped stoma surgery method is needed to reduce tension.

Uncontrollable urinary diversion is often not accepted by patients or parents due to urinary bladder control problems and mucosal eversion complications. Controllable urinary diversion surgery significantly improves the treatment effect of urinary incontinence [21]. The long-term effect of controllable urinary diversion surgery depends on the patency of the skin anastomosis. The output path between the skin and the bladder should be straight, and there should be no sharp bends; at the same time, for those who have never urinated through the urethra or have never inserted a catheter themselves, it is best to place the fistula stoma in the most easily accessible area for CIC. The Mitrofanoff urinary diversion surgery combined with the "VQZ" stoma surgery achieves the controllability of urinary diversion [10, 20], avoids mucosal eversion and urine overflow, facilitates catheterization, and achieves the purpose of controllable urinary diversion.

From the Mitrofanoff urinary diversion surgery, we can see that the newly created urinary path from the skin stoma to the new bladder is very straight. In theory, it is very easy to insert a catheter for catheterization through the new urethra, but because this is a newly made urethra and different from the normal urethra, we need to pay attention to the following points when performing CIC.

8.2 Notes of CIC After Controllable Urinary Diversion Surgery

1. Before discharge, patients, family members, and caregivers should undergo urinary diversion surgery in the hospital CIC procedure training and master the CIC method after urinary diversion surgery.
2. It is best to wear gloves when operating, especially when non-family members are operating. The gloves should be silicone-free, as silicone gloves can easily cause allergies when they come into contact with the skin.
3. There will be two resistances when inserting a catheter into the new bladder through the new urethra via the fistula. One is when passing through the rectus abdominis segment, because this segment is wrapped around the new urethra by the rectus abdominis, similar to the external sphincter of the urethra, and there will be some resistance when passing through. We can generally pass through by slowly applying a little more force. The other is at the submucosal segment of the bladder, which is designed to prevent urine from flowing out of the bladder when the catheter is not inserted, equivalent to the internal sphincter of the urethra. There will also be some resistance when passing through, and we can generally pass through by slowly applying a little more force. This way, the catheter reaches the new bladder.
4. Sometimes the umbilical bladder fistula may become narrow, at which point we can try using a harder catheter to dilate a bit to see if the catheter can be inserted. If not, we need to go to the hospital's urology department for fistula dilation before performing CIC.
5. Sometimes the middle of the new urethra may fold or form a diverticulum, preventing the smooth insertion of the catheter. At this time, we cannot forcibly insert the catheter ourselves, as this could damage the new urethra. We need to go to the hospital's urology department to insert the catheter under endoscopy, and surgery may be required to repair the urethra if necessary.
6. Because the new bladder has weak contraction force, we need to adjust the depth of the catheter and change positions to drain as much urine as possible from the new bladder.
7. Because the new bladder is made from the intestine and the intestinal mucosa secretes mucus, there may sometimes be mucus sediment in the new bladder. We can use a catheter to rinse the bladder with saline to remove the mucus.

8.3 Key Points for Performing CIC After Controllable Urinary Diversion Surgery

1. Prepare supplies. The patient or caregiver should prepare a suitable size and type of catheter, voiding container, cleaning agent, towel, gloves, and other related items as needed. The catheter can be selected according to the size of the skin fistula (generally 10~16 Fr). If the selected catheter cannot be inserted into the skin fistula, a smaller catheter can be used.
2. Choose a comfortable and suitable position. The environment for CIC should be clean and close to the bathroom, and if it's an infant, there should be a diaper changing table. Since the fistula is usually in the navel or upper abdomen, you can choose a sitting, semi-reclining, or lying position. The general principle is as follows: the environment for CIC should be clean and sanitary, and the patient's position should be comfortable and convenient for catheterization. After catheterization, the urine should be easily poured into the toilet.
3. Prepare the consumables on a clean table or flat surface after washing hands with soap and warm water (such as catheters, gloves). You can also prepare the consumables on a clean cloth spread on the table.
4. Patient preparation: For children, they can lie on a flat table or bed and put the catheter into a container, or they can sit on or near the toilet. Adults can stand or sit on the toilet normally.
5. Expose the area and clean: After the patient chooses a suitable position, wipe and clean the

stoma and surrounding area with soap and clean water or non-irritating odor disinfectant two to three times. The order of wiping is to wipe the stoma first and then the skin around the stoma.

6. Gently insert the catheter until urine begins to flow out, and then insert the catheter 3 cm inward. When no urine flows out, you can gently press the bladder area with both hands until no urine flows out of the bladder (Fig. 8.1).
7. After the patient's CIC is finished, gently pull out the catheter, and then wipe and clean the stoma and surrounding area again with soap and clean water or non-irritating odor disinfectant two to three times. The order of wiping is to wipe the stoma first and then the skin around the stoma. Then clean up the used items, wash hands with soap and water, and the CIC is finished.
8. Time interval for CIC after urinary diversion: Within 6 weeks after urinary diversion, the patient needs to carry a catheter to continuously drain the urine in the urine storage bag, and rinse the urine storage bag with saline two times a day. After starting to insert the catheter by yourself, you can change to rinsing twice a week. If the recovery is smooth, on the tenth day, start to clamp the bladder fistula to expand the urine storage bag. The expansion of the urine storage bag starts from half an hour, gradually extending the clamping time. When the patient can tolerate a capacity of 400 mL without pain, remove the tube, and start to insert the catheter by yourself. Initially, the catheter is inserted once every 2 hours, gradually extending to 3 hours, 4 hours, and continuous drainage at night. When the volume of the urine storage bag reaches 600–800 mL, you can stop inserting the catheter at night. To reduce the risk of infection, it is recommended that patients insert the catheter at least every 4–6 hours. Insert the tube once an hour.

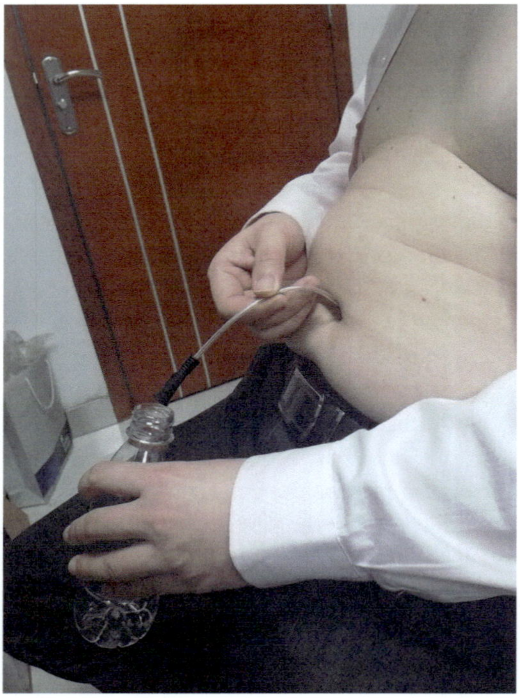

Fig. 8.1 CIC at the umbilical stoma after controllable urinary diversion (see color insert 5)

8.4 CIC Training for Urinary Diversion Patients Before Discharge

Before discharge, patients, family members, and assisting operators who have undergone controllable urinary diversion surgery should receive pre-discharge CIC training. This can enable patients, family members, and assisting operators to correctly and safely perform CIC and improve CIC compliance, thereby reducing the incidence of kidney damage in patients.

Before discharge, patients, family members, and operators are generally trained through videos, meetings, lectures, etc. The training content for adult patients generally includes training on water intake and timing; drinking water each time about 500 mL; drinking water time is from 6 am to 8 pm; each interval is about 3 hours urinate 1 hours after drinking water one time; record for water-containing food, such as soup, porridge, etc.; intermittent catheterization time training; perform CIC before getting up, before meals, and before bed; and perform catheterization 4–6 hours after voiding, to drain the PVR. At the time of discharge, the patient and family members should also be informed of the follow-up time.

8.5 Summary

In summary, in order to successfully perform the new urethra's CIC after controllable urinary diversion surgery, it is necessary to understand the surgical method and understand the shape of the urethra, so that you can perform CIC with confidence. If you encounter difficulties in this process, you can always find a specialist doctor to solve them. In addition, before discharge after urinary diversion surgery, special training should be given to patients and accompanying personnel for CIC, so that patients and accompanying personnel can master the procedure of CIC before discharge, laying the foundation for patients to safely and smoothly complete CIC at home.

References

1. Stein R, Wessel L, Michel MS. Bladder augmentation and urinary diversion in children and adolescents [J]. Urologe A. 2016;55(1):44–52. https://doi.org/10.1007/s00120-015-0006-0.
2. Baradaran N, Stec A, Wang MH, et al. Urinary diversion in early childhood: indications and outcomes in the exstrophy patients [J]. Urology. 2012;80(1):191–5. https://doi.org/10.1016/j.urology.2012.02.028.
3. Flechner SM, Conley SB, Brewer ED, et al. Intermittent clean catheterization: an alternative to diversion in continent transplant recipients with lower urinary tract dysfunction [J]. J Urol. 1983;130(5):878–81. https://doi.org/10.1016/s0022-5347(17)51547-5.
4. Gill IS, Hayes JM, Hodge EE, Novick AC. Clean intermittent catheterization and urinary diversion in the management of renal transplant recipients with lower urinary tract dysfunction [J]. J Urol. 1992;148(5):1397–400. https://doi.org/10.1016/s0022-5347(17)36920-3.
5. Razik A, Das CJ, Gupta A, et al. Urinary diversions: a primer of the surgical techniques and imaging findings [J]. Abdom Radiol (NY). 2019;44(12):3906–18. https://doi.org/10.1007/s00261-019-02179-w.
6. Harper L, Dunand O, Dobremez E. The fallow mitrofanoff [J]. J Pediatr Urol. 2019;15(3):261.e261–4. https://doi.org/10.1016/j.jpurol.2019.02.011.
7. Jonsson O, Olofsson G, Lindholm E, Törnqvist H. Long-time experience with the Kock ileal reservoir for continent urinary diversion [J]. Eur Urol. 2001;40(6):632–40. https://doi.org/10.1159/000049849.
8. Burns R, Speir R, Kern SQ, et al. Early and midterm complications of the continent catheterizable Indiana pouch urinary diversion: a 7-year experience [J]. Urology. 2022;167:229–33. https://doi.org/10.1016/j.urology.2022.04.016.
9. Weibl P, Ameli G, Plank CH, Huebner W. The use of ileocecal pouch with appendix as a urethral substitute in patients who are willing to have a orthotopic bladder replacement – point of technique [J]. Actas Urol Esp (Engl Ed). 2021;45(5):406–11. https://doi.org/10.1016/j.acuroe.2021.04.007.
10. Berrettini A, Rigamonti W, Castagnetti M. Modified VQZ-plasty for the creation of a catheterizable stoma suitable as a neoumbilicus in selected bladder exstrophy patients [J]. Urology. 2008;72(5):1073–6. https://doi.org/10.1016/j.urology.2008.06.061.
11. Stein R, Bogaert G, Dogan HS, et al. EAU/ESPU guidelines on the management of neurogenic bladder in children and adolescent part I diagnostics and conservative treatment [J]. Neurourol Urodyn. 2020;39(1):45–57. https://doi.org/10.1002/nau.24211.
12. Rensing AJ, Szymanski KM, Misseri R, et al. Radiographic abnormalities, bladder interventions, and bladder surgery in the first decade of life in children with spina bifida [J]. Pediatr Nephrol. 2019;34(7):1277–82. https://doi.org/10.1007/s00467-019-04222-w.
13. Barashi NS, Rodriguez MV, Packiam VT, Gundeti MS. Bladder reconstruction with bowel: robot-assisted laparoscopic ileocystoplasty with Mitrofanoff appendicovesicostomy in pediatric patients [J]. J Endourol. 2018;32(S1):S119–26. https://doi.org/10.1089/end.2017.0720.
14. Basavaraj DR, Harrison SC. The Mitrofanoff procedure in the management of intractable incontinence: a critical appraisal [J]. Curr Opin Urol. 2006;16(4):244–7. https://doi.org/10.1097/01.mou.0000232044.03051.aa.
15. De Los Reyes T, Maizels M, Dale R, et al. CEVL interactive – best surgical practices for Open Mitrofanoff Procedure [J]. J Pediatr Urol. 2017;13(3):243–5. https://doi.org/10.1016/j.jpurol.2017.04.006.
16. Famakinwa O, Gundeti MS. Robotic assisted laparoscopic Mitrofanoff appendicovesicostomy (RALMA) [J]. Curr Urol Rep. 2013;14(1):41–5. https://doi.org/10.1007/s11934-012-0294-5.
17. Radojicic ZI, Perovic SV, Vukadinovic VM, Bumbasirevic MZ. Refluxing megaureter for the Mitrofanoff channel using continent extravesical detrusor tunneling procedure [J]. J Urol. 2005;174(2):693–5. https://doi.org/10.1097/01.ju.0000164747.90562.59.
18. Sultan S, Hussain I, Ahmed B, et al. Clean intermittent catheterization in children through a continent catheterizable channel: a developing country experience [J]. J Urol. 2008;180(4 Suppl):1852–5; discussion 1855. https://doi.org/10.1016/j.juro.2008.03.118.
19. Itesako T, Nara K, Matsui F, et al. Clinical experience of the VQZ plasty for catheterizable urinary stomas [J]. J Pediatr Urol. 2011;7(4):433–7. https://doi.org/10.1016/j.jpurol.2010.05.012.

20. Landau EH, Gofrit ON, Cipele H, et al. Superiority of the VQZ over the tubularized skin flap and the umbilicus for continent abdominal stoma in children [J]. J Urol. 2008;180(4 Suppl):1761–5; discussion 1765–6. https://doi.org/10.1016/j.juro.2008.04.070.
21. Stein R, Hohenfellner M, Pahernik S, et al. Urinary diversion--approaches and consequences [J]. Dtsch Arztebl Int. 2012;109(38):617–22. https://doi.org/10.3238/arztebl.2012.0617.

CIC Adjunctive Therapy for SNM Patients

9

Jian-Guo Wen

With the development of medical technology, sacral nerve stimulation (SNS), also known as sacral neuromodulation (SNM), has become another new technology for treating voiding dysfunction. The concept of SNM treatment for voiding dysfunction can be traced back to the 1960s. With the successful application of cardiac pacemakers, people began to try to stimulate other organs of the body through electrical stimulation. In 1979, Schmidt and others conducted animal experiments on SNM in the United States, and in 1981, they initiated a clinical research program on SNM [1]. In Europe, in 1994, SNM was certified by the European community and applied to clinical practice [2]; in the same year, Matzel and others reported the successful experience of SNM in patients with fecal incontinence [3]. In the United States, in 1997, the FDA approved SNM for the treatment of urge incontinence, and in 1999, it was approved for the treatment of frequency-urgency syndrome and urinary retention [2]. Through the continuous efforts and attempts of scholars, in the past decade or so, SNM has undergone tremendous technological updates, including barbed electrodes, intraoperative X-ray fluoroscopy technology, and the application of small stimulators [4]. In 2006, the Interstim II stimulator is used in Europe and America. The volume and weight of the Interstim II stimulator are more than 50% less than those of the Interstim I stimulator, and it can be directly connected to the electrode without the need for extension wires, making permanent implantation simpler and more minimally invasive [5]. As SNM has been successful in treating various refractory urinary disorders, the advantages of this technology have gradually emerged, making more and more urologists begin to pay attention to this technology; thus many indications for CIC have been replaced by SNM, or CIC and SNM are combined to play their respective advantages [6]. The application of SNM in CIC patients can not only increase the patient's ability to urinate autonomously, reduce the patient's PVR, but also extend the interval of CIC, improving the patient's quality of life [7].

Now introduce CIC adjunctive therapy for SNM patients.

9.1 Mechanism of Sacral Nerve Stimulation

SNM, commonly known as "bladder pacemaker," uses interventional technology to continuously apply low-frequency electrical pulses to specific sacral nerves, thereby exciting or inhibiting nerve pathways, regulating abnormal sacral nerve reflex arcs, and thus affecting and regulating the

J.-G. Wen (✉)
Pediatric Urodynamic Center/Department of Urology, First Affiliated Hospital of Zhengzhou University, Zhengzhou, China

J.-G. Wen (ed.), *Progress in Clean Intermittent Catheterization*, Experts' Perspectives on Medical Advances, https://doi.org/10.1007/978-981-97-5021-4_9

bladder and urethra. SNM is a neuroregulation technique that improves the function of target organs innervated by the sacral nerve, such as the anal sphincter and the pelvic floor, thereby achieving therapeutic effects [8].

The storage and voiding functions of the lower urinary tract depend on a series of extremely complex neural reflex regulations of bladder-urethral activities. The brain, brainstem, spinal cord, and peripheral nerves/neural ganglia form a multi-level regulation system through the pelvic nerve, hypogastric nerve, and pudendal nerve to coordinate lower urinary tract activities. The complexity of the neural control of lower urinary tract function also determines the diversity of causes and complexity of treatment [9]. The SNM technique achieves this by inserting a stimulating electrode into the sacral foramen to adhere to the corresponding nerve branches, usually the S3 sacral foramen, to pulse-stimulate the S3 nerve, thereby improving the function of the bladder detrusor, urethral sphincter, and pelvic floor muscles. The mechanism of SNM's impact on lower urinary tract dysfunction is as follows [10].

In patients with non-obstructive urinary retention, SNM can help patients restore pelvic floor muscle function, achieve relaxation of the pelvic floor muscles, and initiate voiding; at the same time, it can inhibit overly strong protective reflexes, close the excitatory effect of the urethra, and promote bladder emptying [11].

In patients with NB, SNM can inhibit preganglionic neurons of the bladder parasympathetic and pelvic nerve efferents to the bladder through pudendal nerve afferents; can activate interneurons in the spinal cord that coordinate bladder and sphincter function, emptying the bladder; and can inhibit overactive bladder reflexes mediated by C fiber conduction pathways [12].

In patients with interstitial cystitis/pelvic pain syndrome, SNM can reduce the overactivity of the pelvic floor muscles, alleviate the symptoms of interstitial cystitis, restore the levels of epidermal growth factor and anti-proliferative factor to normal; block abnormal C fiber activity; and inhibit abnormal micturition reflexes in the spinal cord and above the spinal cord [13].

9.2 Surgical Steps of Sacral Nerve Stimulation

SNM is divided into two stages: the first stage is the external experience therapy of sacral nerve modulation; the second stage is permanent implantation of the sacral nerve stimulator [14]. The external experience therapy stage allows clinicians and patients to understand the clinical effects of the device on the patient. If the patient's various clinical indicators such as daily PVR, daily urine volume, maximum urine volume, and daily voiding times improve by more than 50%, or the patient is satisfied, the permanent stimulation system can be implanted into the body.

External experience therapy stage: The patient takes the prone position, with the lumbar sacral part elevated. Preoperative cross-positioning method is used to locate the S3 nerve foramen and mark it; under local anesthesia, a needle is inserted about 2 cm above the marked point, noting that the puncture needle enters the skin at a 60° angle. When entering the corresponding sacral foramen, there is a feeling of emptiness, then connect to the temporary stimulator, test the patient's motor response and sensory response to confirm whether the puncture site is correct, and X-rays can be taken at any time during the procedure to confirm the position and depth of the puncture needle; after the test is correct, bury the self-fixing electrode, lead the electrode into the subcutaneous fat of one side of the buttock through the subcutaneous puncture channel device, expand the subcutaneous pouch, connect the extension wire to the tail end of the electrode, and the extension wire passes through the subcutaneous tunnel and exits the body surface and is connected to the external stimulation box at the same time; then, according to the degree of symptom improvement during the patient's experience period and the patient's own wishes, decide whether to enter the permanent implantation stage, and use antibiotics after the procedure to prevent infection [3] (Fig. 9.1).

Permanent implantation stage: Under local anesthesia, an incision is made in the upper pouch area of the left buttock, the connection between the electrode wire and the extension wire is found

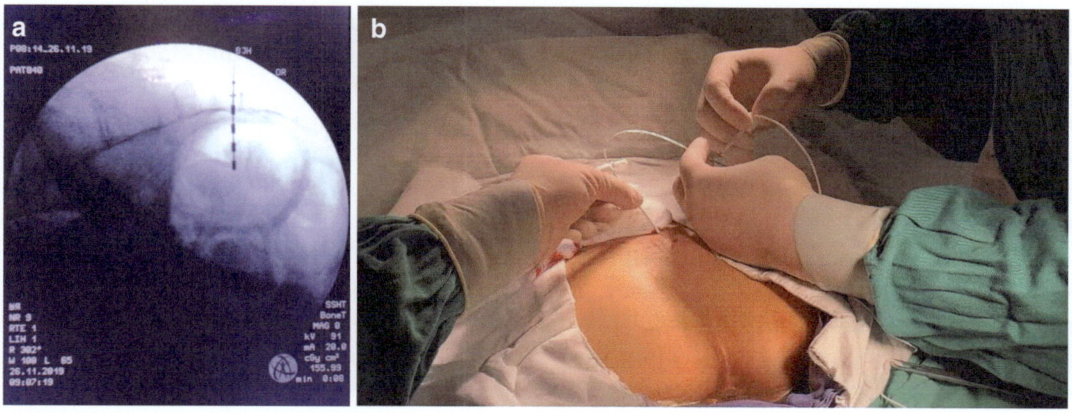

Fig. 9.1 Sacral nerve stimulator puncture position and depth (**a**) and anal response (**b**)

and untied, and the extension wire is pulled out; a pouch is bluntly dilated on the fascia of the incision, the electrode wire is connected to the permanent stimulator, and the wire is placed under the stimulator, noting that the electrode LOGO faces the skin; after the parameters are ideally adjusted, the stimulator is fixed under the pouch, and the incision is closed, and antibiotics are used after the procedure to prevent infection [15].

9.3 Clinical Application of Sacral Nerve Electrical Stimulation

9.3.1 Indications

SNM can be used for various refractory lower urinary tract dysfunctions. The indications currently approved by the US FDA are as follows: (1) refractory urgency urinary incontinence, stubborn urinary frequency, urgency syndrome (also known as refractory OAB) [16, 17]; (2) idiopathic urinary retention [18]; (3) defecation dysfunction, such as fecal incontinence [19]. Refractory means that conservative treatments such as drugs are ineffective or cannot tolerate the adverse reactions of treatment; idiopathic means non-obstructive and non-neurogenic, and the cause is not yet clear.

9.3.2 Relative Indications

Researches have shown that SNM has certain therapeutic effects on NB, pelvic pain syndrome, interstitial cystitis, and chronic constipation, but large sample prospective studies and long-term follow-up are needed to further confirm [20].

9.3.3 Application of CIC and SNM in the Treatment of Patients with Voiding Dysfunction

The clinical symptoms of neurogenic lower urinary tract dysfunction are complex, often combined with intestinal and erectile dysfunction, which brings trouble to the choice and evaluation of treatment. Initially, NB was not considered an indication for SNM. Later studies found that SNM can also achieve good therapeutic effects in NB patients. A systematic review and meta-analysis of SNM treatment of NB was published in the European Urology Journal in 2010 [21]. The article screened 26 independent studies, with a total of 357 patients. The success rate of the trial treatment phase was 68.0%, and the adverse reaction rate was 0; after permanent implantation, the average follow-up was 26 months, the success rate was 92.0%, and the adverse reaction rate was 24.0% [21]. The Department of Urology of Beijing Boai Hospital of China Rehabilitation Research Center, as one of the earliest units to carry out this technology in China, also has rich experience in SNM treatment of NB and has summarized nearly 10 years of experience; a total of 40 NB patients underwent SNM treatment, of which 33 cases were combined with multiple symptoms. After 1–3 weeks of evaluation, the effectiveness rate for frequency and urgency symptoms reached 59.1%, the effectiveness rate for incontinence symptoms was 72.2%, the effectiveness rate for dysuria was 22.2%, and the effectiveness rate for constipation was 68.8%. In the end, 20 patients chose permanent implantation. Among them, not all symptoms of 12 patients with multiple symptoms improved, including 10 patients who had no significant improvement in dysuria and still had more PVR. However, urinary frequency, urgency, urinary incontinence, and constipation improved, and such patients still need CIC to empty urine; only two patients have improved constipation symptoms.

For SNM treatment of NB patients, although some patients have reduced dysuria and PVR, it is only because the urethral resistance has become smaller and Valsalva and Credé maneuver are still needed to assist with urination. Beijing Boai Hospital found that one patient improved ≥50% in urgency incontinence, frequent voiding, urgency, dysuria, and constipation during the test phase, but 1 year later, left bladder ureteral reflux occurred, which was caused by long-term increase in abdominal pressure during voiding. Wyndaele and others [22] reported that more than 40.0% use Valsalva. Patients who perform the action may experience urine reflux. Therefore, sacral nerve stimulation can alleviate urinary incontinence, frequent voiding, urgency, dysuria, and constipation while performing CIC, to avoid VUR caused by long-term Valsalva action, which not only improves the symptoms of NB storage period but also protects the upper urinary tract function with low-pressure voiding. Lombardi G and others [23] reported that in eight cases of incomplete spinal cord injury with urinary retention, after SNM, the amount of urination significantly increased, the number of catheterizations per day significantly decreased, and urodynamic results showed that the upper urinary tract was safe. For some patients with urinary retention, if UDS proves that this method is unsafe for the upper urinary tract after permanent SNM placement, they can also try to empty the urine by CIC. In addition, for patients with NB detrusor overactivity, SNM can significantly reduce the number of urinary urgency and incontinence, reduce bladder pressure, and improve bladder compliance, and these patients can also use SNM combined with CIC to rebuild storage and voiding function.

Xu reported that compared with patients treated with CIC for detrusor weakness, the improvement of voiding frequency, nocturia, PVR, maximum detrusor voiding contraction pressure, and effective detrusor contraction time in patients with detrusor weakness treated with SNM is significantly higher. However, the patients chosen are not those with complete absence of detrusor contraction, some of whom have a certain contraction force in the bladder itself, and the maximum detrusor contraction pressure is improved after SNM treatment, so the PVR is also reduced accordingly. Lombardi G's [24] research found that the poor effect of some patients with urinary retention after SNM may be related to the location of upper motor neuron and lower motor neuron injury. Mid-term and long-term follow-up found that patients with lower motor neuron injury have a significant decrease or complete loss of perineal area perception, leading to the absence of perineal reflex when the bladder responds, resulting in less clinical benefit for these patients after SNM treatment, so these patients are more suitable for emptying the bladder by CIC.

Research [25] has found that among the various symptoms of NB patients, the improvement rate of dysuria during the SNM test phase is significantly lower than that of frequent voiding, urgency, incontinence, and constipation, which is different from the distribution of efficacy in the population of non-neurogenic bladder patients. In non-neurogenic bladder patients, 70–83% of patients with urinary retention can achieve ≥50% improvement [25]. Therefore, the cause of dysuria in NB patients is different from that in non-neurogenic patients. The cause of non-neurogenic urinary retention may be overactivity of the pelvic floor and loss of central control of the pelvic floor. SNM may guide patients to rebuild pelvic floor function and inhibit the protective reflex of the urethra, thereby promoting bladder emptying, rather than directly inducing detrusor contraction. However, the dysuria in patients with NB originates from the coordination disorder of detrusor sphincter and the weakening of detrusor contraction force, so the effect of SNM treatment will be reduced. Whether choosing SNM treatment or CIC, or a combination of both for patients with various urinary functional disorders, clinicians should strictly consider their indications, with the ultimate goal of effectively emptying the bladder, protecting the safety of upper urinary tract, and improving the quality of life.

References

1. De Wachter S, Vaganee D, Kessler TM. Sacral neuromodulation: mechanism of action [J]. Eur Urol Focus. 2020;6(5):823–5. https://doi.org/10.1016/j.euf.2019.11.018.
2. Groen J, Pannek J, Castro Diaz D, et al. Summary of European Association of Urology (EAU) guidelines on neuro-urology [J]. Eur Urol. 2016;69(2):324–33. https://doi.org/10.1016/j.eururo.2015.07.071.
3. Matzel KE, Chartier-Kastler E, Knowles CH, et al. Sacral neuromodulation: standardized electrode placement technique [J]. Neuromodulation. 2017;20(8):816–24. https://doi.org/10.1111/ner.12695.
4. Noblett K, Crowder C. Neuromodulation [J]. Obstet Gynecol Clin N Am. 2021;48(3):677–88. https://doi.org/10.1016/j.ogc.2021.05.018.
5. Spinelli M, Sievert KD. Latest technologic and surgical developments in using InterStim therapy for sacral neuromodulation: impact on treatment success and safety [J]. Eur Urol. 2008;54(6):1287–96. https://doi.org/10.1016/j.eururo.2008.01.076.
6. Liberman D, Ehlert MJ, Siegel SW. Sacral neuromodulation in urological practice [J]. Urology. 2017;99:14–22. https://doi.org/10.1016/j.urology.2016.06.004.
7. Haider MZ, Annamaraju P. Bladder catheterization [M]. Treasure Island: StatPearls Publishing; 2024. Copyright © 2024, StatPearls Publishing LLC.
8. De Wachter S, Knowles CH, Elterman DS, et al. New technologies and applications in sacral neuromodulation: an update [J]. Adv Ther. 2020;37(2):637–43. https://doi.org/10.1007/s12325-019-01205-z.
9. Panicker JN, Fowler CJ, Kessler TM. Lower urinary tract dysfunction in the neurological patient: clinical assessment and management [J]. Lancet Neurol. 2015;14(7):720–32. https://doi.org/10.1016/s1474-4422(15)00070-8.
10. Moore CK, Rueb JJ, Derisavifard S. What is new in neuromodulation? [J]. Curr Urol Rep. 2019;20(9):55. https://doi.org/10.1007/s11934-019-0920-6.
11. Albabtain M, Chughtai B, Cho A, Elterman D. Review of the rechargeable sacral neuromodulation system to treat refractory overactive bladder [J]. Ther Deliv. 2021;12(5):353–62. https://doi.org/10.4155/tde-2021-0007.
12. Averbeck MA, Moreno-Palacios J, Aparicio A. Is there a role for sacral neuromodulation in patients with neurogenic lower urinary tract dysfunction? [J]. Int Braz J Urol. 2020;46(6):891–901. https://doi.org/10.1590/s1677-5538.Ibju.2020.99.10.
13. Tutolo M, Ammirati E, Heesakkers J, et al. Efficacy and safety of sacral and percutaneous tibial neuromodulation in non-neurogenic lower urinary tract dysfunction and chronic pelvic pain: a systematic review of the literature [J]. Eur Urol. 2018;73(3):406–18. https://doi.org/10.1016/j.eururo.2017.11.002.
14. Goldman HB, Lloyd JC, Noblett KL, et al. International Continence Society best practice statement for use of sacral neuromodulation [J]. Neurourol Urodyn. 2018;37(5):1823–48. https://doi.org/10.1002/nau.23515.
15. Luchristt D, Amundsen CL. Strategies for difficult fluoroscopic landmarking during sacral neuromodulation lead placement [J]. Urology. 2023;174:218–20. https://doi.org/10.1016/j.urology.2022.12.029.
16. Blok BFM. Sacral neuromodulation and onabotulinumtoxinA for refractory urge urinary incontinence offer similar success during 2-year follow-up [J]. Eur Urol. 2018;74(1):74–5. https://doi.org/10.1016/j.eururo.2018.03.016.
17. Tilborghs S, De Wachter S. Sacral neuromodulation for the treatment of overactive bladder: systematic review and future prospects [J]. Expert Rev Med Devices. 2022;19(2):161–87. https://doi.org/10.1080/17434440.2022.2032655.
18. Shaker HS, Hassouna M. Sacral root neuromodulation in idiopathic nonobstructive chronic urinary retention [J]. J Urol. 1998;159(5):1476–8. https://doi.org/10.1097/00005392-199805000-00017.
19. Lagares-Tena L, Millán-Paredes L, Lázaro-García L, et al. Sacral neuromodulation in patients with congenital faecal incontinence. Special issues and review of the literature [J]. Tech Coloproctol. 2018;22(2):89–95. https://doi.org/10.1007/s10151-017-1742-5.
20. Thomas T. Sacral neuromodulation for LUTS has promising long-term outcomes [J]. Nat Rev Urol. 2021;18(2):72. https://doi.org/10.1038/s41585-021-00424-w.
21. Kessler TM, La Framboise D, Trelle S, et al. Sacral neuromodulation for neurogenic lower urinary tract dysfunction: systematic review and meta-analysis [J]. Eur Urol. 2010;58(6):865–74. https://doi.org/10.1016/j.eururo.2010.09.024.
22. Wyndaele JJ, Madersbacher H, Kovindha A. Conservative treatment of the neuropathic bladder in spinal cord injured patients [J]. Spinal Cord. 2001;39(6):294–300. https://doi.org/10.1038/sj.sc.3101160.
23. Lombardi G, Nelli F, Mencarini M, Del Popolo G. Clinical concomitant benefits on pelvic floor dys-

functions after sacral neuromodulation in patients with incomplete spinal cord injury [J]. Spinal Cord. 2011;49(5):629–36. https://doi.org/10.1038/sc.2010.176.
24. Lombardi G, Musco S, Celso M, et al. Sacral neuromodulation for neurogenic non-obstructive urinary retention in incomplete spinal cord patients: a ten-year follow-up single-centre experience [J]. Spinal Cord. 2014;52(3):241–5. https://doi.org/10.1038/sc.2013.155.
25. Sanford MT, Suskind AM. Neuromodulation in neurogenic bladder [J]. Transl Androl Urol. 2016;5(1):117–26. https://doi.org/10.3978/j.issn.2223-4683.2015.12.01.

10 Urodynamic Study and Voiding (Catheterization) Diary Are Helpful for Guiding Precise CIC

Jian-Guo Wen

How to individualize the selection of CIC frequency is a problem faced in the process of CIC treatment [1]. Adult patients with good bladder compliance generally perform CIC every 4–6 hours, and both too frequent and too infrequent will increase the chance of infection and injury. However, for patients with poor bladder compliance, in order to ensure the safe catheterization pressure of the bladder (<30 cmH_2O), the frequency of catheterization may need to be increased. If you can urinate on your own (or rely on abdominal pressure/Credé maneuver), if the PVR is less than 100 mL or less than 10–20% of the maximum bladder capacity for a continuous period of time, you can extend the interval of CIC. Whether you want to understand bladder pressure or voiding, you can't do without urodynamic testing and voiding (catheterization) diary [2, 3]. UDS can provide various parameters to help grasp the indications for CIC and guide "precision CIC" and efficacy evaluation [4]. For patients who still have some autonomous voiding function, recording voiding diaries and catheterization diaries in a fixed format can dynamically evaluate the efficacy, which is instructive for precise CIC. The bladder capacity of children of different ages varies greatly, and it cannot be evaluated by the standard of post-void residual (PVR) alone. UDS and voiding (catheterization) diaries are more important for the evaluation of children's CIC.

J.-G. Wen (✉)
Pediatric Urodynamic Center/Department of Urology, First Affiliated Hospital of Zhengzhou University, Zhengzhou, China

10.1 The Guiding Significance of Urodynamic Study for CIC

UDS is divided into non-invasive and minimally invasive types. The uroflowmetry with ultrasound PVR measurement is convenient and can guide the frequency and interval of CIC. Minimally invasive cystometry, pressure/flowmetry (CMG/PFS), etc. can measure the maximum cystometric capacity (maximum cystometric capacity, MCC), bladder compliance (bladder compliance, BC), whether there is detrusor overactivity during filling (detrusor overactivity, DO), weakened detrusor contraction during voiding, etc., to more accurately assess the indications and contraindications of CIC and guide and evaluate the efficacy of CIC [5, 6]. Combined with VUDS, bladder ureteral reflux and detrusor pressure, bladder safe capacity, combined bladder diverticulum, urethral stricture, urethral fistula, and other issues can also be fully evaluated.

The method of using uroflowmetry/PVR measurement to guide CIC is applicable to patients who still have partial autonomous urination function. Free flowmetry is a simple, non-invasive examination method, which can objectively

J.-G. Wen (ed.), *Progress in Clean Intermittent Catheterization*, Experts' Perspectives on Medical Advances, https://doi.org/10.1007/978-981-97-5021-4_10

reflect the voiding process of the lower urinary tract; the flow rate represents the entire emptying process of the bladder, reflecting the function of the bladder, bladder neck, urethra, and urethral sphincter during voiding, and their relationship with each other [7, 8]. The main observation parameters include maximum flow rate, average flow rate, voided volume, voiding time, flow time, and uroflow pattern (cure shape).

It is recommended to use the maximum flow rate combined with voided volume and PVR to report the results of flowmetry, where the flow rate is accurate to 1 mL/s, and the volume is accurate to 1 mL.

The urine remaining in the bladder after voiding is called PVR, and there are many methods for its measurement, such as direct catheterization measurement, color Doppler ultrasound, portable ultrasound measurement, etc. (Figs. 10.1 and 10.2).

The PVR measured immediately after voiding by catheterization (within 5 minutes) is the most accurate, but it must be measured with a measuring cup. The disadvantage of measuring PVR by catheterization is that it is invasive and there is a possibility of urinary system infection caused by catheterization. During urodynamic testing, if bladder pressure measurement is performed, PVR can be measured by catheterization. Abdominal ultrasound measurement of PVR is simple and non-invasive, but it depends on ultrasound equipment [9]. Continuous increase in PVR often indicates an increase in bladder outlet resistance or a decrease in bladder contraction force or both. However, normal PVR does not rule out urethral obstruction and detrusor-sphincter dyssynergia. Therefore, only PVR measurement cannot distinguish whether the PVR originates from detrusor dysfunction or from BOO. Detrusor hypofunction is manifested as a decrease in contraction ability (myogenic decompensation), and in many cases, it is also manifested as poor maintenance of contraction ability. This situation can be primary and idiopathic or secondary to BOO, infrequent voiding, or NB dysfunction [10]. There is usually an

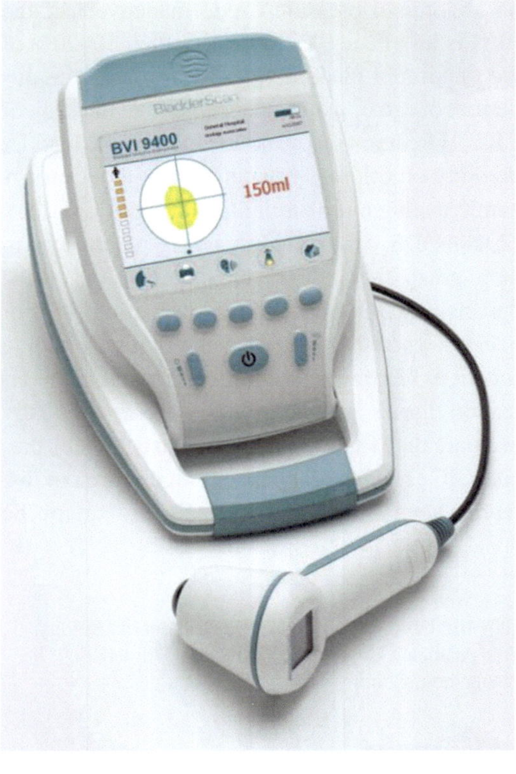

Fig. 10.1 Portable ultrasound measurement device

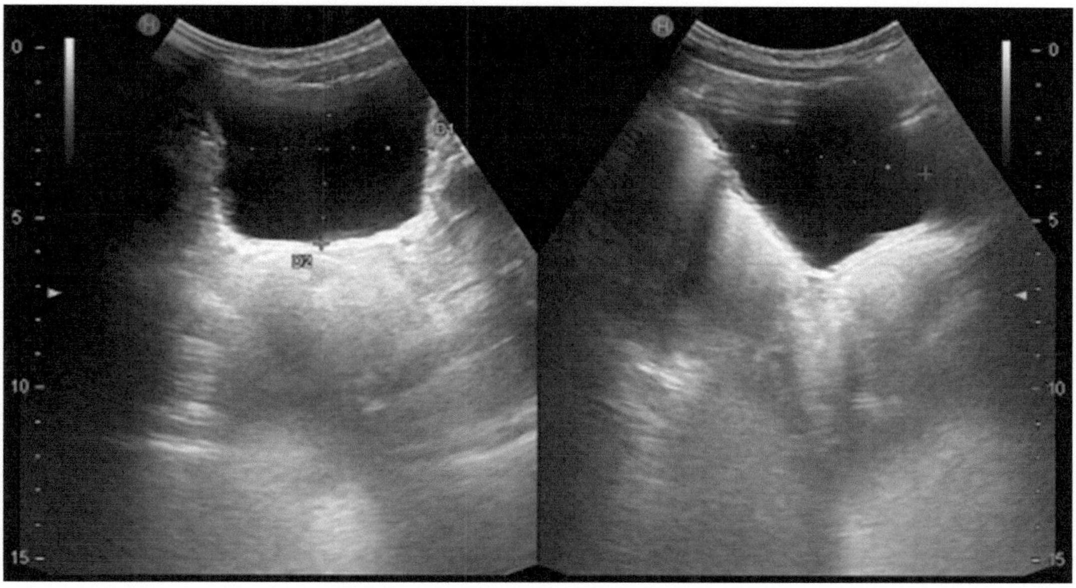

Fig. 10.2 Ultrasonic bladder residual urine measurement

intrinsic correlation between sensory threshold, first voiding sensation, bladder pressure volume, and PVR. For infants, PVR is generally less than 10% of the expected bladder capacity, but individual differences are large. For children aged 4–6 years, PVR > 30 mL or >21% of the expected bladder capacity is abnormal. If PVR > 20 mL or >10% of the expected bladder capacity after secondary voiding, it is considered significantly increased PVR. The PVR of a normal adult is <50 mL or <10% of the expected bladder capacity.

10.2 Cystometry and Pressure/Flow Study to Assess Voiding Dysfunction

Cystometry evaluates bladder storage function through MCC, BC, and other parameters during the storage phase of the bladder [11]. Bladder filling phase abnormalities related to CIC include detrusor overactivity, detrusor hyperfunction, bladder sensation hypersensitivity or loss, MCC too small or too large, BC reduction, filling incontinence, etc., mainly seen in NB, overactive bladder syndrome, NE, and daytime urinary incontinence (DUI) in children.

BC refers to the relationship between bladder capacity and pressure (mL/cmH_2O): the increased capacity when the pressure increases by 1 cmH_2O. It reflects that the bladder wall obtains the maximum capacity with the smallest pressure change. ICS defines it as $C = \Delta V/\Delta P$, where C represents compliance, ΔP represents the increase in pressure, and ΔV represents the increase in bladder capacity when the pressure increases by ΔP. The normal reference value of BC is >20 mL/cmH_2O. The characteristic of a low compliance bladder is that as the bladder capacity increases, the bladder pressure significantly increases. For patients with low compliance bladder (Fig. 10.3), if the filling phase detrusor pressure exceeds 40 cmH_2O, it is high bladder pressure, which can easily cause upper urinary tract damage and hydronephrosis.

Detrusor leak point pressure (DLPP) is the detrusor pressure at the time of leakage during bladder filling in the absence of detrusor autonomous contraction and without abdominal pressure [12]. During bladder filling, due to the decrease in bladder compliance, leakage occurs when the intravesical pressure exceeds the urethral resistance as the filling volume increases. DLPP is mainly used to assess the risk of upper urinary tract damage caused by decreased bladder com-

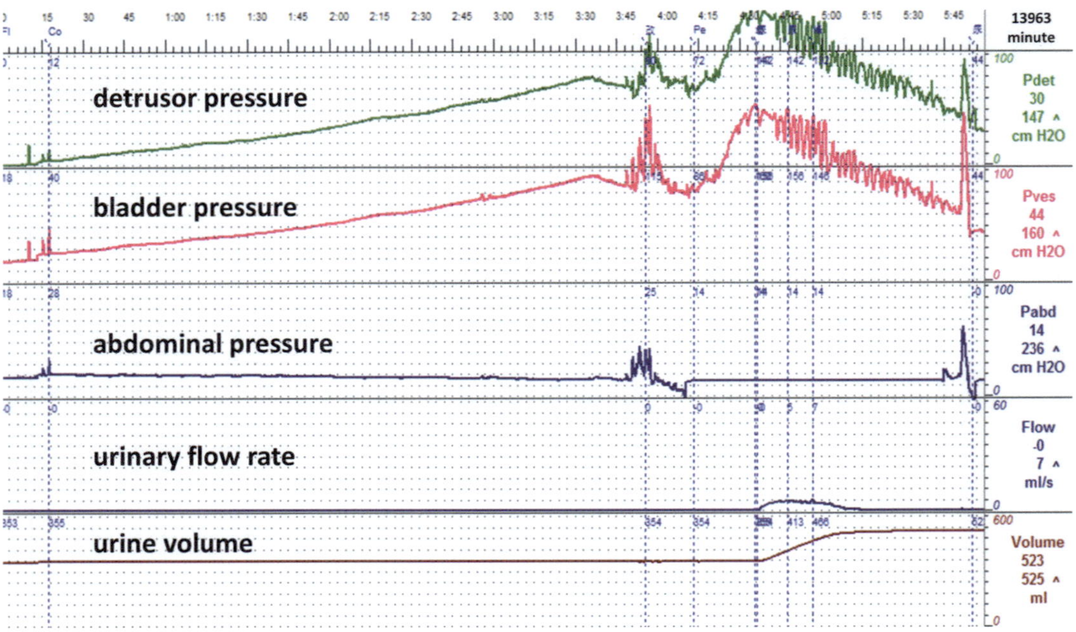

Fig. 10.3 Cystometry shows that the bladder filling end pressure is significantly increased (at the arrow) and the bladder compliance decreased

pliance [13, 14]. The method for measuring DLPP is the patient remains quiet and naturally relaxed during the examination, avoids suppressing voiding and all strenuous actions, and adopts continuous low-speed intravesical infusion (10–20 mL/min) until urine leakage occurs, marking the detrusor pressure at this time. In the absence of detrusor autonomous contraction and changes in abdominal pressure, the bladder capacity when the detrusor pressure during infusion is less than 40 cmH_2O is the safe bladder capacity. The smaller the safe bladder capacity, it means that the time of low pressure in the bladder is shorter, the expansion of the upper urinary tract occurs earlier, the degree of expansion is more serious, or it causes VUR (Fig. 10.4). Therefore, CIC should be performed before the bladder is filled to the maximum safe capacity, and the CIC is adjusted in conjunction with the voiding and catheterization diary; adjust the frequency and interval of time, and adjust the diet and drinking plan.

Pressure flow study (PFS), by measuring the strength of voiding phase detrusor contraction and the dynamic changes of flow rate and detrusor pressure, determines whether there is a weakening of the detrusor contraction and lower urinary tract obstruction [11, 15]. For patients with urinary incontinence, synchronous bladder urethral pressure measurement can be performed if necessary to understand the coordination of the detrusor and the urethral sphincter. Bladder voiding dysfunction is mainly seen in neurogenic detrusor contraction weakness or absence and obstructive diseases such as male prostate hyperplasia, ure-

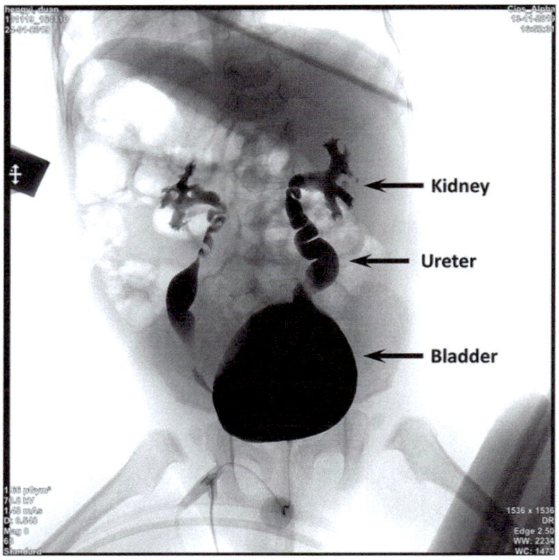

Fig. 10.4 Infant neurogenic bladder VUR

thral stricture, and posterior urethral valve in children. MCC and SBC can guide the timing and frequency of CIC to maximize the protection of the upper urinary tract and ensure that CIC is performed before reaching the safe bladder capacity.

10.3 Video Urodynamic Study of Voiding Function and Urinary Tract Morphological Changes

Video urodynamics (VUDS) refers to the real-time dynamic graphics of the entire urinary tract displayed and recorded on the basis of CMG/PFS, mainly used for evaluation of complex voiding dysfunction, such as DSD, bladder ureteral reflux and hydronephrosis, post-prostate surgery obstruction or incontinence, female voiding difficulty, controllable urinary diversion postoperative review, etc. [16, 17].

Urodynamic parameters related to VUDS include the stability of the filling bladder, bladder sensation, bladder compliance, bladder safety capacity, etc. During voiding, the contraction force of the detrusor and the detrusor pressure at maximum urinary flow rate (PdetQmax) can be recorded. For patients with bladder diverticulum or VUR.

For patients with bladder diverticulum and VUR, it is recommended not to insert too deeply during CIC to avoid causing mucosal injury by inserting the catheter into the diverticulum or inserting it into the ureter through the bladder ureteral entrance [17].

For patients with lower urinary tract obstruction, synchronous X-ray images can also judge anatomical abnormalities, but it is not the only basis for diagnosing obstruction. It should also be judged based on various urodynamic parameters such as free urinary flow rate and PVR. In 1998, the International BPH Advisory Committee recommends that CMG/PFS is currently an effective method to identify lower urinary tract obstruction before invasive treatment or when a diagnosis of obstruction caused by prostate hyperplasia is required. In female with dysuria, 50% have detrusor dysfunction. The most common cause of female lower urinary tract obstruction is mid-to-far urethral obstruction, which can be seen in cases with scar formation or DSD [18].

10.4 Combination of Pediatric Urodynamic Study and CIC

The indications for pediatric UDS include neurogenic voiding dysfunction (spina bifida, meningocele or myelomeningocele, spinal cord schisis, tethered cord syndrome), anorectal malformation-related voiding abnormalities, VUR, urinary incontinence, lower urinary tract obstruction, and unclarified kidney and ureteral hydronephrosis by imaging examination [19, 20].

The pediatric urethra is small, and children often cry and are difficult to cooperate during catheterization, whether it is CIC or carry out UDS, which adds a lot of difficulties [21]. The following points should be noted [22–24]: (1) The expected bladder capacity can be estimated according to age (months). (2) Choose the appropriate size and model of disposable catheter for CIC; for children, 6 and 8 Fr are commonly used. (3) The uncooperation of children may affect the accuracy of urodynamic data. It is recommended to perform multiple uroflowmetry and PVR measurement, and those who need to perform CMG/PFS can appropriately repeat filling to increase accuracy, and try to reduce the interference caused by crying-induced abdominal pressure. (4) Children of different ages need to adjust the frequency of CIC based on expected bladder capacity, flow rate and PVR, bladder safety capacity, etc. If the amount of urine drained each time CIC is above the safe capacity, the frequency of CIC needs to be increased, and the interval time reduced. (5) Weakened detrusor contraction force and increased PVR, DSD, and BOO are all risk factors for upper urinary tract damage. Appropriate treatment measures should be taken as early as possible. It is recommended to perform early CIC after VUDS evaluation.

10.5 Precise Guidance of CIC by Voiding and Catheterization Diary

When performing CIC, it is necessary to accurately record various data in the catheterization diary, such as the amount of water intake (including the types of fluids taken and the number of intakes) and the time and interval of each catheterization, the amount of urine drained each time and whether it is combined with frequent voiding, leakage, hematuria, etc. Adjust the amount of water intake reasonably according to the amount of urine. The child should drink more water evenly to maintain a certain amount of urine production to prevent urinary tract infection, but avoid taking a large amount of fluid in a short time [25, 26].

The voiding diary is widely used in the study of various voiding dysfunctions. It is the simplest and non-invasive examination to assess the function of the lower urinary tract, and it is not restricted by location.

The International Continence Society divides the voiding diary into three types [27]:

1. Micturition time chart: Simply record the number of voiding during the day and night (at least 24 hours).
2. Frequency-volume chart: Record the number of voiding during the day and night (at least 24 hours) and the amount of each voiding; the most important parameters are voiding frequency (day and night), 24 hours urine volume, night and day urine volume ratio, and average urine volume (day and night).
3. Bladder diary: Record the number of voiding, voided volume, occurrence of urinary incontinence, use of urine pads, fluid intake, urgency, degree of urinary incontinence, etc. The 24 hours voiding diary can record the time and amount of water intake, and adjust the amount of water intake appropriately according to the urine volume, and the 24 hours urinary diary is applicable to patients who cannot urinate autonomously or cannot complete voiding through Credé maneuver and calculates indicators such as the total amount of fluid intake in 24 hours, total amount of catheterization, and maximum single catheterization volume.

When recording voiding and catheterization diaries, several indicators can also be integrated into a unified record, and calculate the total amount of fluid intake in 24 hours, total amount of voiding, total amount of catheterization, maximum single voided volume, maximum single catheterization volume, etc. Combining the voiding and catheterization diary, estimate the patient's bladder capacity and PVR, and then perform catheterization and drainage of urine again, and repeatedly verify. To prevent UTI as much as possible, the frequency of catheterization is generally four to eight times per day, which can be adjusted according to the PVR indicators.

References

1. Ghahestani SM, Karimi S. Intermittent catheterization frequency and interval in children: are we clear enough? [J]. Urol J. 2021;18(3):362–3. https://doi.org/10.22037/uj.v18i.6827.
2. Panicker JN. Neurogenic bladder: epidemiology, diagnosis, and management [J]. Semin Neurol. 2020;40(5):569–79. https://doi.org/10.1055/s-0040-1713876.
3. Tudor KI, Sakakibara R, Panicker JN. Neurogenic lower urinary tract dysfunction: evaluation and management [J]. J Neurol. 2016;263(12):2555–64. https://doi.org/10.1007/s00415-016-8212-2.
4. Welk B, Schneider MP, Thavaseelan J, et al. Early urological care of patients with spinal cord injury [J]. World J Urol. 2018;36(10):1537–44. https://doi.org/10.1007/s00345-018-2367-7.
5. Rosier P, Schaefer W, Lose G, et al. International Continence Society Good Urodynamic Practices and Terms 2016: urodynamics, uroflowmetry, cystometry, and pressure-flow study [J]. Neurourol Urodyn. 2017;36(5):1243–60. https://doi.org/10.1002/nau.23124.
6. Panicker JN, Fowler CJ, Kessler TM. Lower urinary tract dysfunction in the neurological patient: clinical assessment and management [J]. Lancet Neurol. 2015;14(7):720–32. https://doi.org/10.1016/s1474-4422(15)00070-8.
7. Xing T, Ma J, Ou T. Evaluation of neurogenic bladder outlet obstruction mimicking sphincter bradykinesia in male patients with Parkinson's disease [J]. BMC Neurol. 2021;21(1):125. https://doi.org/10.1186/s12883-021-02153-4.
8. Wen JG, Djurhuus JC, Rosier P, Bauer SB. ICS educational module: pressure flow study in children [J]. Neurourol Urodyn. 2018;37(8):2311–4. https://doi.org/10.1002/nau.23730.
9. Park YH, Ku JH, Oh SJ. Accuracy of post-void residual urine volume measurement using a portable ultrasound bladder scanner with real-time pre-scan imaging [J]. Neurourol Urodyn. 2011;30(3):335–8. https://doi.org/10.1002/nau.20977.

10. Mcguire EJ. Urodynamics of the neurogenic bladder [J]. Urol Clin North Am. 2010;37(4):507–16. https://doi.org/10.1016/j.ucl.2010.06.002.
11. Drake MJ. Fundamentals of terminology in lower urinary tract function [J]. Neurourol Urodyn. 2018;37(S6):S13–9. https://doi.org/10.1002/nau.23768.
12. Tarcan T, Demirkesen O, Plata M, Castro-Diaz D. ICS teaching module: detrusor leak point pressures in patients with relevant neurological abnormalities [J]. Neurourol Urodyn. 2017;36(2):259–62. https://doi.org/10.1002/nau.22947.
13. Danforth TL, Ginsberg DA. Neurogenic lower urinary tract dysfunction: how, when, and with which patients do we use urodynamics? [J]. Urol Clin North Am. 2014;41(3):445–52, ix. https://doi.org/10.1016/j.ucl.2014.04.003.
14. Kim YH, Kattan MW, Boone TB. Bladder leak point pressure: the measure for sphincterotomy success in spinal cord injured patients with external detrusor-sphincter dyssynergia [J]. J Urol. 1998;159(2):493–6; discussion 496–7. https://doi.org/10.1016/s0022-5347(01)63957-0.
15. Morita T, Kondo S, Tsuchida S. Percutaneous double-lumen catheter for pressure flow study of upper urinary tract [J]. Urology. 1984;24(1):75–6. https://doi.org/10.1016/0090-4295(84)90394-7.
16. Rantell A, Shakir F, Cardozo L. Ambulatory urodynamics monitoring – a video demonstration [J]. Neurourol Urodyn. 2018;37(8):2305. https://doi.org/10.1002/nau.23573.
17. Concodora CW, Reddy PP, Vanderbrink BA. The role of video urodynamics in the management of the valve bladder [J]. Curr Urol Rep. 2017;18(3):24. https://doi.org/10.1007/s11934-017-0670-2.
18. Kuo HC. Videourodynamic characteristics and lower urinary tract symptoms of female bladder outlet obstruction [J]. Urology. 2005;66(5):1005–9. https://doi.org/10.1016/j.urology.2005.05.047.
19. Sager C, Barroso U Jr, Bastos JMN, et al. Management of neurogenic bladder dysfunction in children update and recommendations on medical treatment [J]. Int Braz J Urol. 2022;48(1):31–51. https://doi.org/10.1590/s1677-5538.Ibju.2020.0989.
20. Stein R, Bogaert G, Dogan HS, et al. EAU/ESPU guidelines on the management of neurogenic bladder in children and adolescent part II operative management [J]. Neurourol Urodyn. 2020;39(2):498–506. https://doi.org/10.1002/nau.24248.
21. Sheikh N. Pediatric catheterization protocol [J]. Mymensingh Med J. 2015;24(3):638–48.
22. Selekman RE, Sanford MT, Ko LN, et al. Does perception of catheterization limit its use in pediatric UTI? [J]. J Pediatr Urol. 2017;13(1):48.e41–6. https://doi.org/10.1016/j.jpurol.2016.09.006.
23. Li Y, Wen Y, He X, et al. Application of clean intermittent catheterization for neurogenic bladder in infants less than 1 year old [J]. NeuroRehabilitation. 2018;42(4):377–82. https://doi.org/10.3233/nre-172366.
24. Martins G, Soler ZA, Batigalia F, Moore KN. Clean intermittent catheterization: educational booklet directed to caregivers of children with neurogenic bladder dysfunction [J]. J Wound Ostomy Continence Nurs. 2009;36(5):545–9. https://doi.org/10.1097/WON.0b013e3181b41301.
25. Mitchell B, Curryer C, Holliday E, et al. Effectiveness of meatal cleaning in the prevention of catheter-associated urinary tract infections and bacteriuria: an updated systematic review and meta-analysis [J]. BMJ Open. 2021;11(6):e046817. https://doi.org/10.1136/bmjopen-2020-046817.
26. Wyndaele JJ. Complications of intermittent catheterization: their prevention and treatment [J]. Spinal Cord. 2002;40(10):536–41. https://doi.org/10.1038/sj.sc.3101348.
27. Karamaria S, Ranguelov N, Hansen P, et al. Impact of new vs. old International Children's Continence Society standardization on the classification of treatment naïve enuresis children at screening: the value of voiding diaries and questionnaires [J]. Front Pediatr. 2022;10:862248. https://doi.org/10.3389/fped.2022.862248.

11 The Application of Ultrasound in CIC Cannot Be Ignored

Jian-Guo Wen

With the increasing clarity and resolution of ultrasound images, it leads to various imaging diagnostic methods for detecting cystic or liquid dark area lesions and distinguishing them from solid tumors. Under good contrast conditions, small lesions with a diameter of 2–3 mm can be found. With the continuous innovation of three-dimensional color Doppler ultrasound diagnostic instrument and three-dimensional volume probe and built-in calculation software, both two-dimensional and three-dimensional ultrasound can measure bladder volume in real time and achieve good consistency and repeatability with CT and other imaging examinations.

The commonly used clinical method to monitor changes in bladder volume is urinary system ultrasound examination; its advantage lies in the real-time scanning of the size and cross-sectional morphology of the kidneys, ureters, and bladder; the presence or absence of hydronephrosis, ureteral dilation, bladder wall thickening, and trabecular changes in the bladder; and the simultaneous measurement of bladder volume and PVR. However, as the ultrasound machine is a large-scale professional medical instrument, both machine operation and ultrasound diagnosis require a professional ultrasound physician [1]. Based on this point, the portable bladder volume meter derived from the combination of ultrasound technology and computer technology was born, which is not limited by time, location, and operator. It can measure and evaluate the bladder volume of patients in need anytime and anywhere, and the whole process is simple to operate and short in measurement time and can be completed by clinically trained health-care worker, making routine monitoring of bladder volume in CIC patients possible [2]. Nowadays, portable bladder volume meters are widely used in CIC, NB, posterior urethral obstruction caused by prostate disease, postpartum urinary retention after cesarean section, bladder volume monitoring, and follow-up of patients with pelvic tumor chemotherapy. Therefore, the application of ultrasound in CIC cannot be ignored [3, 4].

J.-G. Wen (✉)
Pediatric Urodynamic Center/Department of Urology, First Affiliated Hospital of Zhengzhou University, Zhengzhou, China

11.1 The Development of the Urinary System and the Basics of Ultrasound Imaging

11.1.1 The Development of the Kidney and Ureter

The embryonic development of the kidney can be divided into three stages, namely, the pronephros, mesonephros, and mesonephros, that appear successively from the neck of the embryo to the pelvis.

J.-G. Wen (ed.), *Progress in Clean Intermittent Catheterization*, Experts' Perspectives on Medical Advances, https://doi.org/10.1007/978-981-97-5021-4_11

1. Pronephros: Occurs at the beginning of the fourth week of embryonic development, located at the 7th to 14th somites on the outside; several transverse cell cords (pronephric tubules) are formed from the head end of the nephrogenic cord, the inner end opens to the embryonic coelom, and the outer end extends to the tail and connects into a longitudinal pronephric duct. The pronephros degenerates at the end of the fourth week of embryonic development, but most of the pronephric duct is retained and continues to extend to the tail, developing into the mesonephric duct.
2. Mesonephros: Occurs at the end of the fourth week. After the pronephros, located at the 14th to 28th somites on the outside, many transverse tubules, called mesonephric tubules, occur successively from head to tail in the mesonephric ridge, the outer end of the mesonephric tubules, and the pronephric duct extending to the tail merge into the mesonephric duct. The tail end of the mesonephric duct enters the cloaca. By the end of the second month of the embryo, most of the mesonephros degenerates, leaving only the mesonephric duct and a small portion of the caudal mesonephric tubules, which form a part of the reproductive duct in males and only a small portion in females, becoming accessory tissues such as ovaries and fallopian tubes.
3. Metanephros: Develops into the permanent kidney. At the beginning of the fifth week of embryonic development, when the mesonephros is still developing, the metanephros begins to form. From the 11th to 12th week, the metanephros begins to produce urine, which continues throughout the fetal period. The urine is discharged into the amniotic cavity and constitutes the main component of the amniotic fluid. The metanephros originates from two different parts, the metanephrogenic blastema and the ureteric bud, both of which originate from the mesoderm.
4. Ureteric bud: The ureteric bud is a blind tube that grows dorsolaterally from the end of the mesonephric duct near the cloaca. It extends toward the dorsal and cranial side of the embryo, growing into the mesodermal tissue at the end of the mesonephric ridge. The ureteric bud branches repeatedly, evolving into the ureter, renal pelvis, calyces, and collecting tubules.
5. Metanephrogenic blastema: The metanephrogenic blastema is produced by the mesodermal tissue at the end of the mesonephric ridge under the induction of the ureteric bud. The peripheral part of the metanephrogenic blastema evolves into the renal capsule, while the inner part forms multiple cell clusters, which attach to both sides of the ends of the arcuate collecting tubules. These epithelial cell clusters gradually differentiate and, as the ends of the collecting tubules continue to grow and branch into the cortical superficial layer, successively induce the formation of superficial renal units in the metanephrogenic blastema. As the metanephros occurs on the side of the mesonephric ridge, the original position of the kidney is relatively low. With the growth of the embryonic abdomen and the extension of the ureteric bud, the kidney gradually rises to the lumbar region.

11.1.2 The Development of the Bladder and Urethra

During the fourth to seventh week of embryonic development, the urorectal septum separates the cloaca into the dorsal rectum and the ventral urogenital sinus [5]. The urogenital sinus is divided into three sections: (1) The upper section is larger and develops into the bladder. Its apex is connected to the urachus, which degenerates into a fibrous cord from the umbilicus to the top of the bladder before birth, called the median umbilical ligament. The left and right mesonephric ducts open into the bladder, respectively. As the bladder enlarges, a section of the mesonephric duct below the beginning of the ureter also enlarges and gradually merges into the bladder, becoming part of its posterior wall, so the ureter and mesonephric duct open into the bladder, respectively. (2) The middle section of the urogenital sinus is quite narrow, remains tubular, forms the urethra in females, and becomes the prostatic and membranous part of the urethra in males. Due to factors such as the kidney's migration toward the cranial side and the continued growth of the mesonephric duct, the opening of the ureter moves to the outer upper side, while the opening of the mesonephric duct in males moves down to the prostatic part of the urethra; in females, the part that enters the urethra will degenerate. (3) The lower section forms the spongy part of the urethra in males, while in females, it expands into the vestibule of the vagina.

11.2 Ultrasonography of Urinary System: Procedure and Normal Manifestations

11.2.1 Ultrasound Equipment and Probe Frequency

Color Doppler ultrasound diagnostic device, built-in convex array probe, and linear array probe [6]. Frequency of convex array probe: for adults it is 3.5–3.75 MHz; for children it is 3–5 MHz, and for linear array probe, it is 5–10 MHz.

11.2.2 Examination Method

The examinees are all examined in a quiet state. Both adults and children are recommended to use convex array and combine with linear array; first use the convex array probe to scan the entire kidney, ureter, and bladder; combine with the linear array probe when detecting focal lesions and small lesions, to improve its lesion resolution [7]. The convex array probe is the first choice when measuring bladder volume and PVR, which is conducive to better enveloping the bladder boundary and accurate measurement. When the ultrasound machine has built-in three-dimensional volume software and probe, it can further switch to the three-dimensional mode, adjust the volume sampling frame size and pitch angle to cover the entire bladder, dynamically collect the bladder volume data, and measure the three-dimensional volume.

11.2.2.1 Examination Position

Common positions for kidney examination: supine or lateral position, through the side of the waist; prone position, through the back, continuous scanning in longitudinal and transverse sections. Common positions for bladder examination: supine position, above the pubic bone through the abdominal route; lithotomy position, through the long axis of the urethra, continuous scanning in longitudinal and transverse sections.

11.2.2.2 Preparation Before Examination

No special preparation is generally required before kidney examination [8]. Drink enough water to fill the bladder before examining the ureter and bladder.

11.2.3 Ultrasound Performance

Kidney contour line: It is composed of renal fascia and fat inside and outside the fascia. It usually appears as a continuous, smooth strong echo band surrounding the entire kidney.

Renal parenchyma: Located between the renal sinus and the renal contour line, it appears as a low echo, surrounding the renal sinus echo; the normal adult renal parenchyma thickness is about 1–2 cm variably (Fig. 11.1). The renal parenchyma is divided into two parts: (1) renal medulla, also known as renal pyramid, appears as an oval or conical shape radiating around the renal sinus echo; the echo intensity is lower than the renal cortex echo; (2) renal cortex surrounds the outer layer of the renal medulla echo, and a part of it extends between the renal cone echoes; the echo intensity is slightly higher than the renal medulla echo, and the normal renal cortex thickness is about 8–10 mm [9].

Renal sinus: The echo of the renal sinus is a combination of the echoes of various anatomical structures in the renal sinus, including the renal pelvis, renal calyx, blood vessels, and fat tissues, also known as the collecting system echo. The renal sinus usually appears as an elliptical high echo area, located in the center of the kidney. The sonogram section passes through the renal hilum,

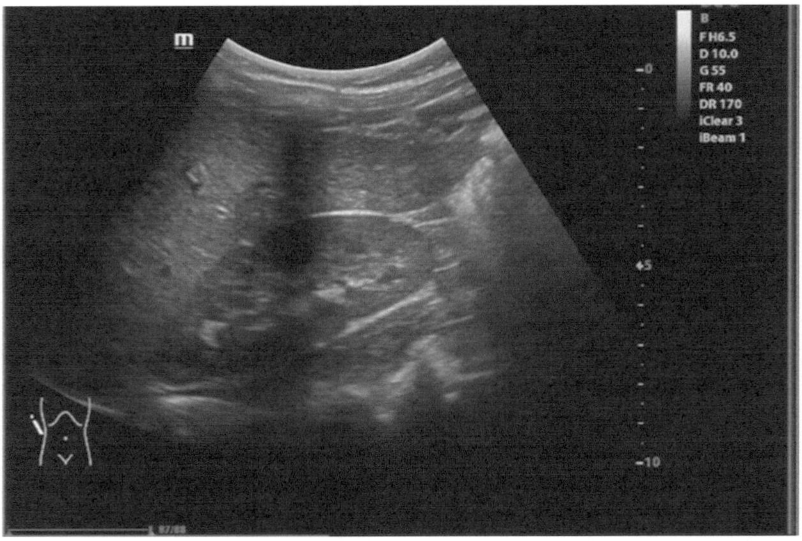

Fig. 11.1 Normal kidney ultrasound (right longitudinal section—coronal section)

and the renal sinus echo extends toward the renal hilum, continuing with the renal contour line.

When there is fluid in the renal pelvis and renal calyx, the renal sinus echo shows a no echo dark area in the middle. Normal kidneys can have no echo areas when drinking a lot of water, bladder filling, taking antispasmodic drugs, or during the fetal period. The diameter of physiological renal pelvis separation is usually less than 1 cm, without renal calyx expansion.

When the renal pelvis separation is greater than 1 cm, combined with renal calyx dilation, hydronephrosis should be considered. In addition, when the difference in length between the two kidneys exceeds 1 cm, structural abnormalities of the kidney should be considered, which are common in unilateral duplicated kidneys, bilateral renal pelvis malformations, and underdeveloped kidneys.

Renal vessels: Color Doppler ultrasound can display the main renal artery, segmental artery, interlobar artery, arcuate artery, down to the interlobular artery in the cortical surface of the kidney, and its accompanying various levels of renal veins [10]. Pulsed Doppler can measure the blood flow spectrum of each segment of the renal artery. The normal renal artery blood flow spectrum shows a rapidly rising systolic single peak, followed by a slowly declining diastolic flat extended segment. There is a small sharp peak before the contraction peak of the main renal artery and its large branches, with a notch between the two peaks. The normal renal vein blood flow spectrum shows a negative low level, flat extended line; the main renal vein spectrum shows a negative double peak, which can fluctuate with respiration and the pulsation of the inferior vena cava.

Ureter: The ureter is a slender muscular tube with rhythmic peristalsis. Normal ureter ultrasound is difficult to display, and the display rate increases when the ureter dilates. The junction of the ureter and renal pelvis, the junction with the bladder, and the intramural segment of the bladder are the common sites for congenital stenosis, malformation, and stone obstruction. When ultrasound examination shows hydronephrosis, bladder wall thickening and trabeculation, urethral dilation, and clinical suspicion of stones, congenital ureteral stenosis, VUR, etc., a complete and continuous scan from the kidney to the bladder along the ureteral route is required to avoid missed diagnosis.

Bladder: The urine in the bladder is displayed as a no echo area. The bladder mucosal echo is located at the junction with the urine and appears as a strong echo or high echo. When the bladder is well filled, it appears as a continuous and smooth high echo band. When the bladder is not filled enough, the mucosal echo can appear

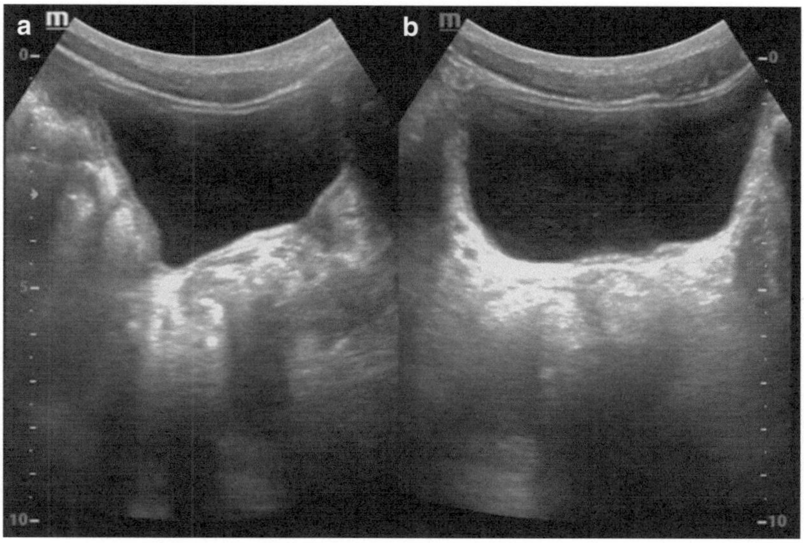

Fig. 11.2 Normal bladder sonogram. (**a**) Longitudinal section, (**b**) cross section

uneven. The bladder muscle layer is displayed as a medium echo or low echo, surrounding the periphery of the mucosa. The normal bladder wall thickness is 1–3 mm, thin when the urine is filled and thick when emptied (Fig. 11.2). Most of the newborn bladder is located in the abdominal cavity and gradually descends with age, reaching the pelvic floor and approximating adults during adolescence.

11.3 Ultrasound Manifestations of Bladder Emptying Disorder Diseases

Bladder emptying disorder diseases are the main targets of CIC treatment, commonly seen in children with congenital spina bifida, spinal meningocele, sacral dysplasia, spinal tumors, meningitis, cerebral palsy, anorectal malformations and other NB functional disorders and lower urinary tract symptoms, enuresis, and other non-neurogenic bladder functional disorders [11]. In adult patients, it is commonly seen after pelvic tumor surgery, BOO, excessive inhibition of reflex hyperactivity by anticholinergic drugs, and bladder enlargement surgery [12].

The clinical manifestations of bladder emptying disorder diseases are mainly abnormal voiding caused by storage dysfunction and emptying dysfunction. Storage dysfunction can manifest as frequent voiding, urgency, urinary incontinence, etc., and emptying dysfunction can manifest as difficulty urinating, increased PVR, etc. The European Association of Urology recommends: newborns with NB caused by congenital spinal cord and spinal deformities such as spina bifida and spinal meningocele should start CIC treatment as soon as possible after birth, and other patients diagnosed with NB due to spinal tumors, meningitis, cerebral palsy, trauma, and anorectal malformations should also start CIC treatment immediately after diagnosis. Previous research and clinical application have confirmed that early treatment can avoid irreversible serious consequences such as decreased bladder compliance, abnormal bladder capacity, VUR, hydronephrosis, renal scarring, renal fibrosis, etc. due to high bladder pressure. In all NB patients, it is recommended to use ultrasound as the first choice of imaging examination to monitor bladder wall thickening and morphological changes, bladder volume changes, bladder diverticula and trabeculae formation, stones, VUR, hydronephrosis, bladder wall and renal blood supply, etc. during the entire process of CIC and conservative treatment, disease monitoring, and follow-up [13].

11.3.1 Ultrasound Equipment and Probes, Examination Methods, Examination Positions and Preparations

As previously described, in the normal ultrasound manifestations of the urinary system.

11.3.2 Ultrasound Manifestations

Ultrasound images of patients with bladder emptying disorders can show persistent or progressively worsening hydronephrosis, ureteral dilation, bladder abnormalities, and urethral obstruction images.

Kidney: The ultrasound image of hydronephrosis shows separation of the renal collecting system, dilation of the renal pelvis and calyces, and thinning of the renal parenchyma. Mild hydronephrosis shows normal kidney size and dilated renal pelvis, accompanied by mild calyx dilation and normal renal parenchyma echo [14]. Moderate hydronephrosis shows enlarged kidney, dilated renal pelvis and calyces, and slightly thinned renal parenchyma (Fig. 11.3). Severe hydronephrosis shows the kidney is significantly enlarged, the renal pelvis and calyces are significantly dilated, and the renal parenchyma is very thin. Color Doppler ultrasound shows that the blood flow signal of the hydronephrotic renal parenchyma is less than that of the normal kidney. When hydronephrosis is unilateral, compared with the healthy side kidney, pulse Doppler can show that the resistance index (RI) of the affected side kidney is significantly increased, and the blood flow velocity and RI of the renal arteries on both sides are asymmetrical.

Ureter: When bladder emptying disorder is not treated in time, effectively chronic urinary retention, further increase in PVR, and long-term high pressure in the bladder lead to VUR. Ultrasound can show unilateral or bilateral dilation of the ureter, which may be accompanied by peristalsis. When combined with urinary system infection, it can show thickening of the ureteral wall, decreased echo, and dense dot-like low echo in the lumen (Fig. 11.4).

Bladder: In the early stage of the disease, the ultrasound image can show rough and unsmooth bladder wall, decreased or increased bladder capacity, and increased PVR in the bladder [15]. In the middle and late stages of the natural course of the disease, as the fibrosis of the bladder becomes more severe, it can show irregular thickening of the bladder wall, trabecular and small room changes, and formation of pseudodiverticula (Fig. 11.5).

When clinically suspecting bladder voiding disorder and performing ultrasound examination,

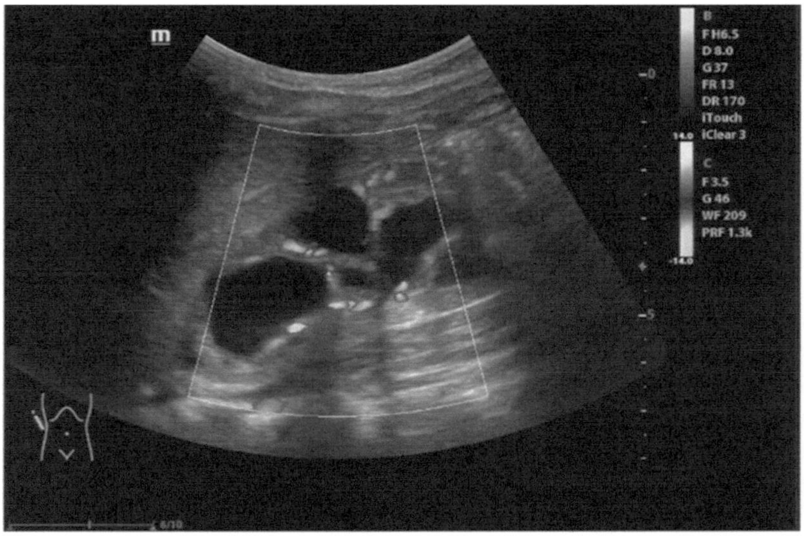

Fig. 11.3 Moderate hydronephrosis ultrasound image of the right kidney (right coronal section Doppler image)

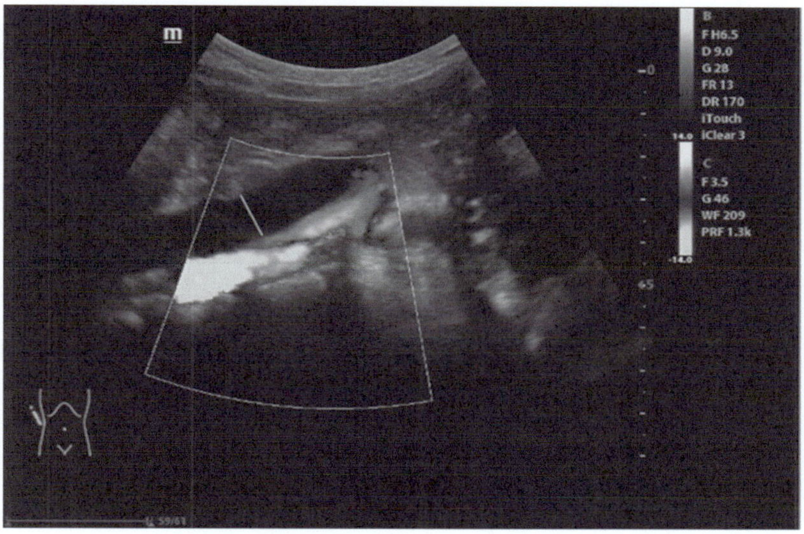

Fig. 11.4 Right ureter dilation ultrasound image (longitudinal section of the ureter Doppler image). The solid line is the anterior and posterior diameter of the dilated ureter

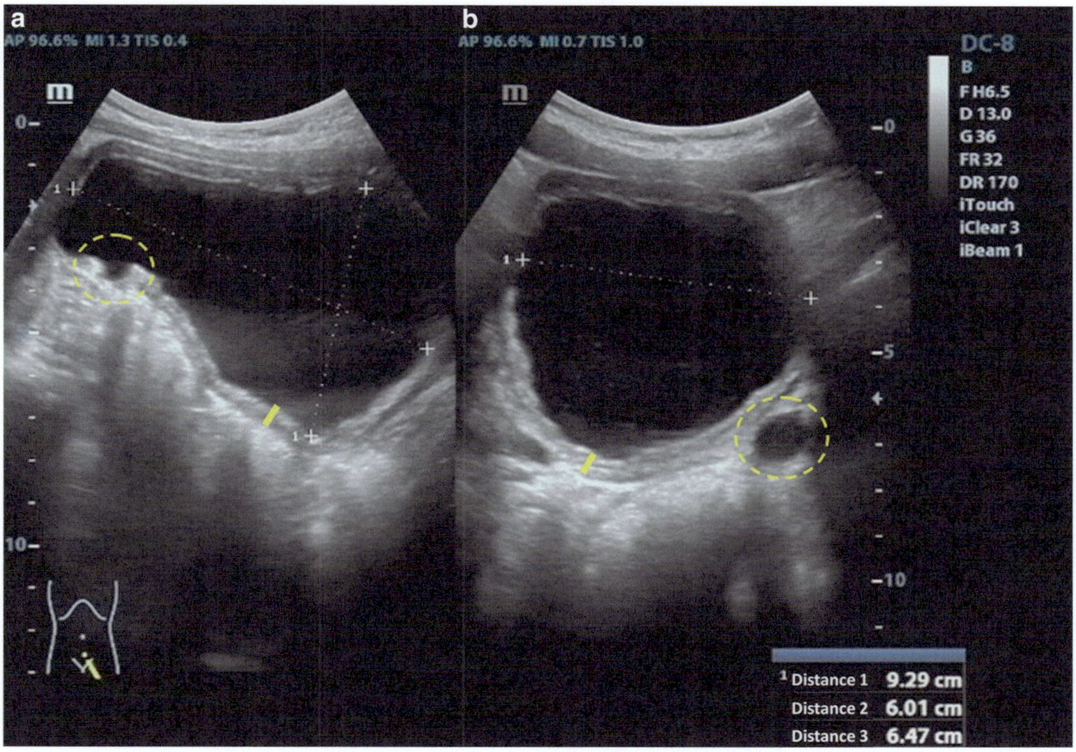

Fig. 11.5 Bladder voiding disorder bladder sonogram, showing how to measure bladder volume (two-dimensional ultrasound—ellipsoid formula). (**a**) The longitudinal section of the bladder shows thickening and roughness of the bladder wall (solid line) and formation of bladder diverticulum (dashed ellipse). (**b**) The cross section of the bladder shows thickening and roughness of the bladder wall (solid line) and dilation of the left ureter (dashed ellipse)

it is necessary to first combine the medical history; understand whether there are congenital spina bifida, spinal meningocele, anorectal malformation, spinal and pelvic and urethral trauma history, etc.; and differentiate it from pelvic tumors, urethral valves, prostate hyperplasia, and other obstructive lesions causing bladder, bilateral kidney, and ureter sonogram abnormalities [16].

11.4 Methods and Precautions for Ultrasound Measurement of Bladder Capacity and Post-voided Residual

11.4.1 Ultrasound Equipment and Probe, Examination Method, Examination Position and Preparation

The equipment, examination method, and preparation for ultrasound measurement of bladder capacity and PVR are the same as the normal ultrasound performance of the urinary system mentioned earlier.

The position for ultrasound measurement of bladder capacity and PVR is supine position, supra-pubic abdominal approach. Convex array probe, frequency: adults 3.5–3.75 MHz, children 3–5 MHz [17].

11.4.2 Method and Principle of Ultrasound Measurement of Bladder Capacity and PVR

The safe capacity of the bladder is measured by ultrasound at the time of the strongest urge to urinate before voiding, and the PVR is measured immediately after voiding. There is no ideal formula for the method of measuring bladder capacity and PVR in clinical practice. The most widely used are the estimation by the ellipsoid formula after measuring the three diameters of the bladder under two-dimensional ultrasound and the application of three-dimensional ultrasound volume method.

Two-dimensional ultrasound—ellipsoid formula: That is, assuming that the bladder is close to an ellipsoid when it is filled, the ellipsoid formula is used to calculate the bladder capacity and PVR.

This method is easy to operate, but due to the certain irregularities and individual differences in human bladder morphology, especially when there are trabecular changes and bladder diverticulum, there are certain errors in the results. During the measurement, the patient is in the supine position, the supra-pubic abdominal approach; the maximum cross-sectional image measures the bladder transverse diameter and thickness, and the maximum longitudinal section image measures the bladder length. The measurement formula is $V = 0.532 \times d_1 \times d_2 \times d_3$, where V is the bladder capacity or PVR and d_1, d_2, and d_3 are the three diameters of the bladder.

Three-dimensional ultrasound volumetric method: Three-dimensional volumetric ultrasound uses a two-dimensional ultrasound transducer to quickly deflect in the pitch angle direction using a mechanical motor, or a matrix electronic probe to obtain volumetric sound images at a frequency of more than 25 frames per second, then applies virtual organ computer-aided analysis technology to geometrically envelope the boundary of the bladder mucosa and quickly calculates the volume measurement method automatically. The accuracy, repeatability, and sensitivity of three-dimensional ultrasound quantification of organ volume are superior to two-dimensional ultrasound. Currently, three-dimensional color ultrasound machines used in clinical applications can complete the measurement of three-dimensional bladder volume after being equipped with a three-dimensional volume probe and built-in volume measurement software.

11.4.3 Precautions for Ultrasound Measurement of Bladder Capacity and PVR

The following points should be noted for ultrasound measurement of bladder capacity and PVR:

1. Patients with chronic urinary retention may have excessive bladder filling. When the bladder envelope is incomplete, the depth of the sampling frame can be adjusted, and the wide-view imaging function of the instrument can be used for correction. When collecting bladder cross-sectional and longitudinal images for volume measurement, the bladder should be completely enveloped as much as possible.
2. Intestine gas can easily cover the top of the bladder, making the measurement value of the bladder's vertical diameter smaller, affecting the accuracy of the measurement results. This can be corrected by using the method of pressing the probe to push away the intestinal gas.
3. When measuring the bladder diameter, the pressure on the longitudinal and cross-sectional surfaces must be the same to avoid errors.
4. Some CIC patients can still urinate on their own. When applying for a clinical measurement of PVR to judge the recovery of autonomous voiding function, it should be noted that when the bladder is overfilled, the measurement value of the PVR is often too large. It is necessary to combine the medical history and communicate with the patient whether they feel they have urinated completely. If necessary, it can be measured again after the next voiding. In addition, when determining the treatment effect and following up the PVR, the same calculation method must be used; otherwise, it may lead to misguidance.

11.4.4 Clinical Significance of Ultrasound Measurement of Bladder Capacity and PVR

Results of the recent studies [18], through retrospective analysis and follow-up of 97 cases of congenital spina bifida caused to NB children, show about 17.5% (17 cases) of the 97 children needed bladder augmentation due to high bladder pressure and bladder ureteral reflux, most children can achieve treatment effects comparable to bladder augmentation through CIC and conservative treatment, while spina bifida, VUR, and high bladder pressure are the most important independent risk factors for long-term bladder augmentation surgery. For such patients, it is recommended to use ultrasonography to monitor bladder capacity, PVR, bladder morphology, and upper urinary tract conditions. Ultrasonic measurement of bladder capacity and PVR has good consistency with the actual bladder capacity measured by catheterization, and it is non-invasive; has no risk of urinary tract infection; is economical; can be monitored in real time, especially for some patients with partial autonomous voiding CIC, ultrasonic measurement of bladder capacity, PVR, and combined with urine flowmetry; can real-time assess the recovery of the bladder; provide a reference for reducing or increasing the number of catheterizations; and help improve the overall accuracy of treatment.

11.5 The Application of Portable Bladder Capacity Measuring Instrument in CIC

With the development of imaging technology and the increasing refinement of clinical needs, portable ultrasound bladder capacity measuring instruments suitable for non-professional ultrasound technicians are widely used in multiple clinical fields [19]. The bladder capacity measuring instrument, also known as the bladder measuring instrument or bladder scanner, is based on modern acoustics and ultrasound principles, imaging technology, and computer automatic plane measurement technology; it can quickly and accurately estimate the urine volume in the bladder and provide a reliable basis for CIC, and the procedure is simple; the measurement time is short; it is not restricted by time, location, and operators; it can measure and evaluate patients anytime and anywhere; and clinical medical staff can complete it after qualified training.

11.5.1 The Detection Position and Probe of the Bladder Capacity Measuring Instrument

Supine position, above the pubic bone through the abdominal route. The instrument is equipped with a convex array probe, and the handle of the probe is equipped with a measurement start button (Fig. 11.6).

11.5.2 The Detection Position, Detection Method, and Principle of the Bladder Capacity Measuring Instrument

When using a bladder measuring instrument for volume measurement, the patient is usually in the supine position, above the pubic bone through the abdominal route. First, the maximum cross-sectional image of the bladder shows the bladder filling state. When the bladder cavity shows anechoic urine filling, the measurement start button of the probe is activated, and its probe can emit and receive ultrasound waves and continuously automatically scan. At 180°, multiple cross-sectional images of the bladder are obtained, the bladder contour is manually outlined, and through image processing, a three-dimensional image is simulated to calculate the bladder volume. After the patient urinates, the measurement mode is restarted in the same position, and the instrument automatically calculates the PVR in the bladder.

11.5.3 Accuracy of the Bladder Capacity Meter

A large number of validations have been carried out on the accuracy and repeatability of the bladder capacity meter. Previous studies have shown that the volume measured by the portable three-

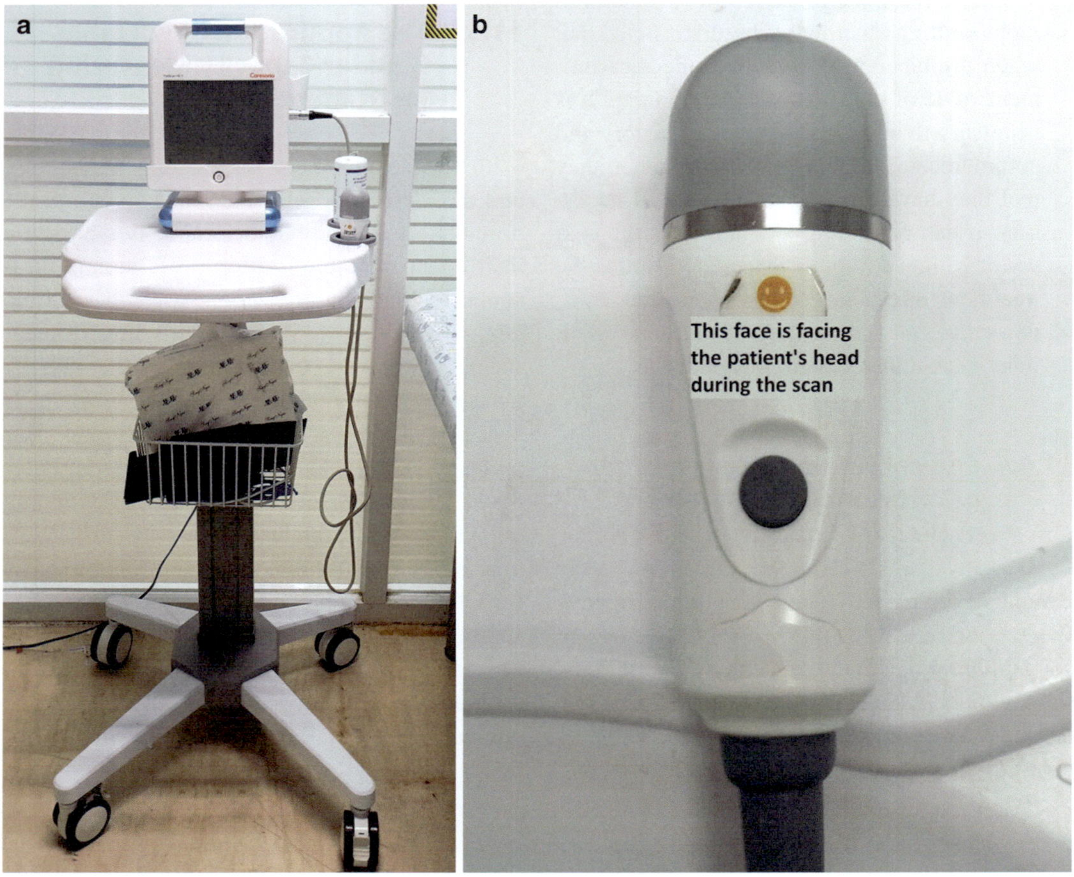

Fig. 11.6 Portable bladder capacity measuring instrument. (**a**) Instrument equipment, (**b**) probe

dimensional ultrasound bladder capacity meter and the three-dimensional ultrasound system measuring the bladder volume of normal people has a significant correlation with the actual capacity of the bladder. The bladder capacity meter can accurately, timely, objectively, and non-invasively measure the bladder volume of patients. The portable ultrasound bladder capacity meter provides a practical and economical method for real-time monitoring of bladder capacity in clinical practice, which helps to improve the accuracy and effectiveness of CIC patient treatment.

11.5.4 Precautions for the Use of Bladder Capacity Meter in CIC

The bladder scanner is operated by trained and skilled clinical medical staff. By monitoring the patient's bladder capacity at any time, it guides CIC interval time, especially for patients with partial autonomous voiding ability; it can assess the ability of partial autonomous voiding of CIC patients, helping patients catheterize before reaching unsafe bladder capacity, preventing excessive bladder expansion and muscle damage to the bladder, reducing the occurrence of urinary system infections, and finding suitable catheterization time points for CIC patients. It promotes the recovery of bladder function in patients and provides reference for reducing or increasing catheterization frequency [19].

When adult patients use the bladder capacity meter to guide CIC treatment and monitor the bladder urine volume <300 mL or below 50% of the safe capacity, catheterization can be delayed; if the bladder urine volume is 300–500 mL, continue to give CIC as usual; if the bladder urine volume is >500 mL, immediate catheterization should be given. For children, the frequency of catheterization is adjusted based on the previously monitored safe bladder capacity and actual urine volume [20]. Moreover, it is necessary to adjust the drinking plan effectively based on the measurement results of the bladder capacity meter and the actual catheterization volume, and urge to drink according to the plan, to protect the function of the bladder and upper urinary tract.

11.5.5 Clinical Significance of Ultrasound Bladder Capacity Meter in CIC

Previous domestic and foreign research and clinical application results show that the bladder capacity meter has high reliability, non-traumatic, simple procedure, high timeliness, and other advantages for the measurement of bladder capacity and PVR, which can be used for CIC. The patient's adjustment and monitoring of intermittent catheterization frequency and timing provide a reliable basis, alleviating the patient's pain and reducing the occurrence of complications, and it is recommended to use in the clinical care and disease management of CIC-treated patients [21].

References

1. Vigil HR, Hickling DR. Urinary tract infection in the neurogenic bladder [J]. Transl Androl Urol. 2016;5(1):72–87. https://doi.org/10.3978/j.issn.2223-4683.2016.01.06.
2. Abrams P, Cardozo L, Fall M, et al. The standardisation of terminology in lower urinary tract function: report from the standardisation sub-committee of the International Continence Society [J]. Urology. 2003;61(1):37–49. https://doi.org/10.1016/s0090-4295(02)02243-4.
3. Timberlake MD, Kern AJ, Adams R, et al. Expectant use of CIC in newborns with spinal dysraphism: report of clinical outcomes [J]. J Pediatr Rehabil Med. 2017;10(3–4):319–25.
4. Nazarko L. Intermittent self-catheterisation: past, present and future [J]. Br J Community Nurs. 2012;17(9):408, 410–412. https://doi.org/10.12968/bjcn.2012.17.9.408.
5. Alamo L, Gengler C, Hanquinet S, et al. Prenatal magnetic resonance imaging of complex female genitourinary system abnormalities, what the fetal medicine specialist needs to know [J]. Prenat Diagn. 2023;43(1):84–94. https://doi.org/10.1002/pd.6264.
6. Fiori G, Pica A, Sciuto SA, et al. A comparative study on a novel quality assessment protocol based on image analysis methods for color Doppler ultrasound diagnostic systems [J]. Sensors (Basel). 2022;22(24):9868. https://doi.org/10.3390/s22249868.

7. Desmots F, Fakhry N, Mancini J, et al. Shear wave elastography in head and neck lymph node assessment: image quality and diagnostic impact compared with B-mode and Doppler ultrasonography [J]. Ultrasound Med Biol. 2016;42(2):387–98. https://doi.org/10.1016/j.ultrasmedbio.2015.10.019.
8. Reisinger N, Ahmed N. The ultrasound-augmented physical exam for nephrologists: beyond the kidney [J]. Adv Chronic Kidney Dis. 2021;28(3):191–2. https://doi.org/10.1053/j.ackd.2021.10.005.
9. Jeong JY, Kim SH, Lee HJ, Sim JS. Atypical low-signal-intensity renal parenchyma: causes and patterns [J]. Radiographics. 2002;22(4):833–46. https://doi.org/10.1148/radiographics.22.4.g02jl04833.
10. Stock KF. [Ultrasound diagnostics of renal blood vessels and transplant kidney] [J]. Radiologe. 2009;49(11):1040–7. https://doi.org/10.1007/s00117-009-1873-4.
11. Panicker JN. Neurogenic bladder: epidemiology, diagnosis, and management [J]. Semin Neurol. 2020;40(5):569–79. https://doi.org/10.1055/s-0040-1713876.
12. Di Benedetto P. Clean intermittent self-catheterization in neuro-urology [J]. Eur J Phys Rehabil Med. 2011;47(4):651–9.
13. Kaye IY, Payan M, Vemulakonda VM. Association between clean intermittent catheterization and urinary tract infection in infants and toddlers with spina bifida [J]. J Pediatr Urol. 2016;12(5):284.e281–6.
14. Partik BL, Stadler A, Schamp S, et al. 3D versus 2D ultrasound: accuracy of volume measurement in human cadaver kidneys [J]. Investig Radiol. 2002;37(9):489–95. https://doi.org/10.1097/01.Rli.0000023573.59066.43.
15. Bright E, Oelke M, Tubaro A, Abrams P. Ultrasound estimated bladder weight and measurement of bladder wall thickness--useful noninvasive methods for assessing the lower urinary tract? [J]. J Urol. 2010;184(5):1847–54. https://doi.org/10.1016/j.juro.2010.06.006.
16. Marzuillo P, Guarino S, Capalbo D, et al. Interrater reliability of bladder ultrasound measurements in children [J]. J Pediatr Urol. 2020;16(2):219.e211–7. https://doi.org/10.1016/j.jpurol.2019.12.015.
17. Rademakers KL, Van Koeveringe GA, Oelke M. Ultrasound detrusor wall thickness measurement in combination with bladder capacity can safely detect detrusor underactivity in adult men [J]. World J Urol. 2017;35(1):153–9. https://doi.org/10.1007/s00345-016-1902-7.
18. López Pereira P, Martinez Urrutia MJ, Lobato Romera R, Jaureguizar E. Should we treat vesicoureteral reflux in patients who simultaneously undergo bladder augmentation for neuropathic bladder? [J]. J Urol. 2001;165(6 Pt 2):2259–61. https://doi.org/10.1016/s0022-5347(05)66179-4.
19. Ghani KR, Pilcher J, Rowland D, et al. Portable ultrasonography and bladder volume accuracy--a comparative study using three-dimensional ultrasonography [J]. Urology. 2008;72(1):24–8.
20. Diéguez I, March JA, Costa-Roig A, et al. Analysis of the predictive capacity of the clinical variables that indicate the performance of voiding urosonography in the study of vesicoureteral reflux in children [J]. Arch Esp Urol. 2022;75(8):693–9. https://doi.org/10.56434/j.arch.esp.urol.20227508.100.
21. Corona LE, Lee T, Marchetti K, et al. Urodynamic and imaging findings in infants with myelomeningocele may predict need for future augmentation cystoplasty [J]. J Pediatr Urol. 2019;15(6):644.e641–5.

12 CIC Process Cannot Ignore Effect Evaluation

Jian-Guo Wen

For CIC, a patient self-management treatment method, regular follow-up, and guidance should be provided to improve patient compliance and timely solve related problems. The timely follow-up and guidance of health-care worker to patients are crucial for improving patient compliance and quality of life [1]. Before carrying out CIC, an assessment of the patient is needed to grasp the indications and decide whether to use CIC and which method, interval time, etc. After carrying out CIC, use different methods at different times to evaluate the effects and deficiencies, which is beneficial to change and adjust the number of CIC, the method, etc. Therefore, the CIC process cannot ignore the effect evaluation. Here we introduce how to accurately evaluate the effect of CIC and its clinical significance.

12.1 Health Education Prior to CIC Assessment

For patients who need to implement CIC, the responsible nurse or doctor first explains the relevant knowledge of CIC and the importance of implementing CIC to the patient in simple and understandable language, teaches the patient or family members the method of catheterization, and explains the precautions during the procedure process.

When the patient first starts to self-catheterize, the nurse supervises every step of the catheterization and gives timely guidance on the problems that exist in the procedure process [2]. For patients with low cultural level and poor acceptance and memory, a clean catheterization process chart is distributed to deepen the patient's impression [3]. The patient is instructed to keep a daily voiding diary, which includes daily drinking situation, amount of each self-voiding, leakage amount, catheterization time, catheterization amount, etc., in order to observe the recovery of bladder function.

Drinking plan: includes control of drinking volume, drinking time, and catheterization interval time [4]. According to the patient's lifestyle, fluid replenishment, and fluid and functional training time, a drinking plan timetable is made for the patient, with a daily drinking volume of 1500–2000 mL.

Try not to drink water after 20:00 to avoid excessive bladder expansion affecting the patient's sleep. The drinking volume includes all fluids, such as milk, soup, and juice. If the above fluids have been consumed, the corresponding amount should be deducted. One to two days before performing clean intermittent catheterization, the patient should be taught to drink water according to the drinking plan. The patient must follow the drinking plan during the preparation

J.-G. Wen (✉)
Pediatric Urodynamic Center/Department of Urology, First Affiliated Hospital of Zhengzhou University, Zhengzhou, China

J.-G. Wen (ed.), *Progress in Clean Intermittent Catheterization*, Experts' Perspectives on Medical Advances, https://doi.org/10.1007/978-981-97-5021-4_12

for intermittent catheterization and during the intermittent catheterization [5]. Water is evenly consumed in each time period within 24 hours to avoid excessive bladder expansion due to inability to urinate or incomplete voiding, damaging the function of each organ of the urinary system.

Clean hand washing: 1–2 days before self-intermittent catheterization, prepare hand washing supplies, and teach the family members of paraplegic or quadriplegic patients to wash their hands according to the clean hand washing step chart and which is one of the key procedures to prevent urinary system infection [6]. The patient or family members must wash their hands carefully, with a hand washing time of more than 5 minutes.

Vahter and others believe that cognitive decline does not affect the ability to learn CIC, but the length of time for teaching patients CIC has a significant impact on compliance, with a minimum teaching time of 1 hour, especially for initial teaching [1].

The following questions can be used to evaluate whether training in CIC has been successful for the patient.

1. What is CIC?
2. List three conditions that may require CIC.
3. What is the recommended standard frequency for performing CIC?
4. What should be included in the Rx table?
5. What should be considered when choosing a supplier?
6. What are the three items that need to be included in the "Letter of Medical Necessity" (LMN)?
7. List three potential problems and suggest what measures should be taken to solve them.
8. What are the three symptoms of a urinary tract infection?
9. List five areas that need to be assessed to determine the patient's readiness to learn.
10. What measures should be suggested if no urine flows out after the catheter is inserted?
11. List one emergency situation that needs to be monitored in patients with spinal cord injuries.
12. What size of catheter is most commonly used by ostomy patients?
13. Describe the general anatomy of the urinary tract.

12.2 Assessment of CIC

Follow up with patients in a convenient way, such as by phone, WeChat, email, etc., to guide them in their subsequent treatment. When following up with patients, first ask about their medical history in detail to understand if there are any comorbidities that may affect the treatment outcome.

During the follow-up process before and after the start of CIC, both renal function and urodynamic bladder function should be assessed [7]. After starting CIC, follow up in the outpatient clinic at 2 weeks, 1 month, and 3 months and then once a year thereafter. Visit the clinic at any time if complications occur. For mature adults, the frequency of urinary system ultrasound follow-ups can be extended to once every 3 years; as long as the urodynamic status of the bladder does not change (such as needing to increase the frequency of CIC to alleviate symptoms of urinary incontinence or an increase in the frequency of urinary tract infections), there is no need for further urodynamic testing [3]. These young people should be closely followed up to ensure that they continue to maintain good CIC habits, and they should be regularly checked to detect any urinary tract infections or stone formation.

12.2.1 Assessment of Renal Morphology and Function

The bladder pressure of patients with NB is higher during both the storage and voiding phases, which further leads to urine reflux to the renal pelvis, resulting in hydronephrosis. It is worth mentioning that due to the increase in PVR in the bladder, bacteria can easily proliferate, leading to recurrent urinary system infections. The reflux to the renal tissue can lead to delayed renal development, renal scarring, and ultimately end-stage renal failure. Therefore, it is very important to assess renal function before and after CIC [8].

Imaging examination: Including ultrasound, urinary tract plain film, urography, MRI, CT scans, etc.

Ultrasound: Ultrasound can determine the degree of hydronephrosis and the atrophy of the renal cortex [9]. It is simple, easy to perform, and non-invasive and should be the preferred evaluation method [10]. Mild hydronephrosis: the shape and size of the kidney are mostly normal, the thickness and echo of the renal parenchyma are normal, and the renal collecting system is separated by 2–3 cm. Moderate hydronephrosis: the kidney volume is slightly increased, the shape is full, the parenchyma is slightly thinned, the renal columns are not clear, the renal pelvis and calyces are obviously dilated, and the renal collecting system is separated by 3–4 cm. Severe hydronephrosis: the kidney volume is increased, the shape is abnormal, the parenchyma is significantly thinned or cannot be displayed, and the entire kidney area is a liquid dark area [9]. There are compressed linearly separated renal columns in between, arranged in a radial pattern; each dark area is interconnected, and the entire image is very similar to a color palette.

Urinary tract plain film: X-ray examination has important value for the evaluation of kidney shape, can see the contour of the enlarged kidney due to hydronephrosis, and can also find the formation of urinary tract stones.

Urography: Early venous urography can see the dilation of the renal calyces and pelvis and the disappearance of the calyx mouth or cystic display; when renal function is reduced, the renal parenchyma display time is prolonged, and the display is unclear; at this time, high-dose delayed imaging can obtain better imaging effects [11]. When the kidney is not clearly displayed in venous urography, retrograde pyelography can be performed, which can often obtain clearer images of hydronephrosis. But this method of examination has the risk of causing infection, and strict aseptic procedure and the use of antibiotics must be ensured during retrograde catheterization.

MRI: Magnetic resonance hydrography has unique advantages in the diagnosis of hydronephrosis and can replace retrograde pyelography. MRI can clearly show the shape, size, and position of both kidneys and is significantly better than ultrasound in displaying the fine structure of the kidney, volume measurement, etc. It has the advantages of being non-invasive, safe, radiation-free, no contrast agent allergy, and no operator skill problems, and urine is a natural contrast agent, which is also suitable for patients with renal function damage.

Although MRI also has relative disadvantages, such as relatively high examination costs and longer examination time, etc., but considering comprehensively, MRI is still widely used in the examination of hydronephrosis, and in hospitals with conditions, it even becomes the preferred imaging examination method.

CT: CT can clearly show the degree of hydronephrosis and the atrophy of the renal parenchyma and has certain value for the objective evaluation of renal function.

Laboratory tests: Including routine urine tests, urine creatinine and urea nitrogen tests, serum creatinine tests, etc.

Routine urine test: Collect fresh urine for examination, preferably mid-stream urine. It can also be obtained through catheterization. Routine urine tests include color, transparency, specific gravity, pH, qualitative protein and glucose, as well as microscopic examination after centrifugal sedimentation; the latter includes cellular components in urine (red blood cells, white blood cells, epithelial cells, and urinary cast), various microorganisms and crystals, etc. Normal fresh urine is light yellow, clear, and transparent, with a specific gravity between 1.003 and 1.030; pH around 6.5 (5.0–8.0); qualitative tests for protein, glucose, ketones, bilirubin, and nitrite all negative; microscopic examination shows 0–3 red blood cells/HP; 0–5 white blood cells/HP, generally no tubules. Abnormal routine urine tests can initially indicate pathological conditions, such as an increase in white blood cells is common in urinary tract infections, which can be used to detect whether the patient has a urinary system infection after performing CIC.

Urine creatinine and urea nitrogen: The normal values are urine creatinine 0.7–1.5 g/24 h and urea nitrogen 9.5 g/24 h. When acute nephritis or renal insufficiency occurs, the content of urine creatinine decreases, an increase in urea nitrogen indicates an increase in tissue decomposition metabolism, and a decrease is seen in renal insufficiency and hepatic parenchymal disease.

Serum creatinine: Creatinine is mainly filtered by the glomerulus, not reabsorbed by the renal tubules; the renal tubules can secrete a small amount when blood creatinine increases, but the amount is negligible, so this method can be used clinically to measure glomerular filtration function. Normal blood creatinine is 1–2 mg/dL (88–177 mmol/L); the higher the serum creatinine value, the worse the kidney function; the two are directly proportional.

CIC, as the first choice for emptying the bladder, can improve the quality of life on the one hand and solve incontinence and voiding problems; another important aspect is to prevent kidney damage. During the filling period, the pressure of the detrusor continues to rise at the end of bladder filling, the ureter refluxes, the urine entering the bladder from the upper urinary tract is obstructed, the kidney pressure rises, the kidney will be damaged and dilated, even causing hydronephrosis, ureteral hydronephrosis, and renal fibrosis, leading to renal failure; performing CIC treatment can keep the bladder in a continuous low-pressure state, protecting kidney function [12]. Before and after performing CIC using imaging examinations and laboratory tests can effectively evaluate the patient's kidney morphology and function; observe the degree of hydronephrosis, urine creatinine, serum creatinine, and other indicators is better than before CIC, which is of great significance for the evaluation of CIC effects.

12.2.2 Urodynamic Study

VUDS is the gold standard for diagnosing and assessing bladder function in patients with NB [13]. It can objectively evaluate bladder function during the filling and voiding phases and is the only method that can objectively evaluate lower urinary tract function. VUDS is the combination of bladder pressure, flow rate, and morphology imaging.

12.2.2.1 Uroflowmetry

Uroflowmetry refers to the method of using a uroflowmeter to measure and record the speed, time, and corresponding urine flow curve of urine discharged from the urethra [14]. The formation of urine flow is the final result of the following processes: detrusor contraction, bladder neck opening, urethral urine transmission, and pelvic floor activity. Generally speaking, the description of urine flow should be carried out from two aspects: the rate of urine flow and the urine flow curve. The urine flow curve can be continuous or intermittent. The flowmetry refers to the volume of urine flowing out of the body through the urethra per unit time, expressed in milliliters per second (mL/s). Attention should be paid to the effects of voided volume, patient environment and position (supine, sitting or standing), bladder filling method, use of diuretics, and the way of using catheters (through the urethra or above the pubic bone) on the flow rate.

The voided volume is the total amount of urine discharged through the urethra; the maximum flow rate is the maximum measured urine flow rate; the average flow rate is the voided volume divided by the voided time [15]. Only when the urine flow is continuous and there is no terminal urine dripping, the calculation of the average flow rate is meaningful. The urine flow time refers to the actual time when the measurable urine flow appears, and the maximum flow rate time refers to the time from the start of voiding to the maximum urine flow rate. When measuring urine flow time and average urine flow rate, the mode of voiding should be explained. To determine whether urine flow is normal, in addition to the maximum urine flow rate, it is also necessary to refer to the shape of the urine flow curve.

Uroflowmetry is a simple, non-invasive examination method, which can objectively reflect the voiding process of the lower urinary tract; the flow rate represents the entire emptying process of the bladder, reflecting the function of the bladder, bladder neck, urethra, and urethral sphincter during voiding, as well as their relationship with each other. It is worth mentioning that some patients who cannot urinate autonomously are not suitable for uroflowmetry, but these patients may recover some autonomous voiding function after a period of CIC treatment.

After treatment, it is possible to reassess the effect of CIC treatment by performing uroflowmetry; for some patients who were able to void autonomously before CIC treatment, it is recommended to perform partial CIC treatment and perform uroflowmetry before and after treatment to observe the recovery of bladder function.

Portable uroflowmeter: Uroflowmetry can only be performed in medical institutions, and many patients find it difficult to keep continuous records due to physical or other reasons [16]. The advent of the portable uroflowmeter eliminates this obstacle. The portable uroflowmeter is a conveniently portable small electronic scale, integrated with high-precision, high-performance analog signal processing components. The electronic scale is disk-shaped, small in size, light in weight, and accurate in weighing data; it has an automatic sensing switch, which can timely power off when not in use to extend the usage time. The middle of the electronic scale is a magnet structure, used to fix the measuring cup with metal. After the patient urinates, the measuring cup filled with urine can be placed on the electronic scale to get the voided volume and time, stored in the electronic scale. And the relevant data is sent to the smartphone through the built-in Bluetooth communication device. After downloading the software on the smartphone, in addition to receiving the voiding information transmitted by the electronic scale regularly, it can also save the data in the phone and realize the display of the voiding diary, the generation of voiding statistical reports, and the input of drinking water information through the graphical interface programming. The software can also establish a network connection with the hospital central server through the mobile phone wireless communication network and regularly send the patient's voiding information and drinking water information to the server. The server automatically stores it, establishes the patient's personal medical record, and generates voiding information reports and charts for the patient in real time. Doctors can directly access the central server through the network to obtain the patient's voiding statistical reports, analysis charts, trend charts, weight bar charts, etc., to help doctors analyze the condition and cause of the disease. By using this system, it can collect the patient's daily urination time, urination volume, drinking time, drinking volume, and sleep and wake-up time. Based on the above information, the patient's total daily urination times, day and night urination times, urine volume, and nocturnal urine weight can be counted, and the patient's daily average indicators can be counted weekly. When the patient's daily average urination times or nocturnal urine weight exceeds the preset parameters, it can be displayed in different colors.

12.2.2.2 PVR Measurement

The PVR refers to the volume of urine remaining in the bladder at the end of voiding [17]. It reflects the interaction between the bladder and the urethral outlet during voiding. The time for measuring PVR should be controlled within 5 minutes after voiding. Continuous PVR increase often suggests increased bladder outlet resistance or weakened bladder contraction or both. Lack of PVR cannot rule out urethral obstruction and detrusor-sphincter dysfunction. Infant PVR is generally less than 10% of bladder capacity, but individual variation is large. Normal children's PVR is generally less than 10 mL and is unrelated to age, gender, and maximum bladder capacity. For adult patients, PVR greater than 50 mL is usually considered abnormal, and further investigation should be considered.

Before starting to measure the PVR, the patient must feel as comfortable as possible, have a normal urge to urinate, adopt the most ideal voiding posture, and have a private voiding environment, so that the patient can accept that this voiding is completely natural and habitual. PVR can be measured through a catheter or ultrasound. Among them, the transurethral catheterization method is considered the "gold standard" for PVR determination. To ensure complete bladder emptying, the catheter needs to be slowly inserted and withdrawn from the urethra, and it can also be gently rotated. However, catheterization is an invasive procedure after all, and there are still many inaccuracies, so it should only be performed when necessary and followed up by urodynamic testing in the future. Ultrasound determination of PVR has the advantages of noninvasiveness, acceptable relative accuracy, and economic convenience, so it is most suitable for PVR determination after simple flowmetry.

The formation of PVR is caused by low detrusor function activity or BOO, so simple PVR determination lacks specificity and cannot distinguish whether the PVR originates from detrusor function abnormalities or from BOO [18]. Detrusor function decline is manifested as a decrease in contraction ability (muscle-originated decompensation), and in many cases, it is also manifested as poor ability to maintain contraction. This situation can be primary and idiopathic, but it is often secondary to BOO, low frequency of urination, or neurogenic bladder dysfunction. The flow rate curve can be completely normal, but it usually weakens or disappears as the bladder empties. The sensory thresholds in the bladder mucosa and urethra often abnormally increase, manifesting as an increase in the first voiding sensation and bladder pressure volume values. There is usually a weak correlation between sensory thresholds, the first voiding sensation, bladder pressure volume, and PVR. The urethral sphincter electromyogram (EMG) usually shows abnormalities, while the response time of the sacral nerve reflex is usually normal.

The ultrasound evaluation of NB has been widely carried out in clinical practice. It is mainly used for PVR determination, bladder wall thickness, and morphology evaluation. Various causes of NB can cause voiding disorders and thus cause a series of corresponding functional and structural changes, resulting in corresponding clinical symptoms and imaging manifestations. Ultrasound examination shows that the bladder wall is rough or thickened to varying degrees; bladder muscle trabeculae and small chambers are formed; bladder volume changes; bladder diverticula of different degrees are formed; the internal urethral orifice is dilated, showing a funnel-shaped change, ureter dilation and hydronephrosis, urinary system stones or secondary infections, etc. It usually takes a long time from the onset to the occurrence of the above complications. If they can be found and treated early, they can reduce the occurrence of the above complications. Determining PVR in patients with NB is an important means to evaluate the degree of disease development. We suggest that patients should determine the PVR before and after CIC treatment, so as to judge the recovery of bladder function, evaluate whether CIC treatment is effective, and thus further guide the treatment of the disease.

Bladder capacity meter (portable ultrasound): CIC is usually performed four to six times a day according to doctor's orders. CIC, due to the lack of a good method to determine the amount of urine in the bladder, is performed on the patient regardless of how much urine is in the bladder at the specified time. This time-based catheterization method can lead to unnecessary catheterization (too little urine in the bladder) and increased frequency of catheterization or too much urine in the bladder not being drained in time, leading to bladder overdistension. Unnecessary CIC can increase the incidence of urinary tract infections, and repeated bladder overdistension can also lead to active infections in the bladder and cause damage to the detrusor. Some studies have compared the bladder capacity measured by a bladder capacity meter with the gold standard (catheterization method). There is a clear linear correlation between the two sets of data, and the difference between 75.5% of the measurements and the actual catheterization volume is within ±50 mL, which is acceptable for guiding CIC. The measurement of PVR can provide an important reference for assessing the recovery of bladder function after CIC treatment, evaluating the effect of CIC treatment, and the bladder capacity meter can also provide convenience for patients to self-assess, which can be used to guide accurate catheterization, reduce unnecessary catheterization, and thus reduce CIC-related complications.

12.2.2.3 Cystometry

Cystometry is the recording of pressure during the uniform filling process of the bladder. The method of reflecting bladder function in relation to volume is usually represented by a bladder pressure-volume curve. It is used to evaluate bladder capacity, compliance, detrusor function, central nervous system control of detrusor reflex, and bladder sensory function during filling. Combined with voiding pressure-flow measurement, it has more clinical value. Bladder pressure-volume measurement estimates and judges the following functions of the bladder through some measured parameters: bladder sensation, detrusor activity, bladder compliance, bladder volume, and urethral function.

Bladder Sensation

Normal bladder sensation: The first desire to void (FD) of a normal bladder appears when the bladder is filled to about 50% MCC, normal voiding sensation (ND) appears at about 75% MCC, and strong desire (SD) appears at about 90% MCC.

Abnormal bladder sensation: (1) Increased bladder sensation, also known as bladder hypersensitivity (BHS), defined as early FD (below one third of the maximum bladder capacity), normal ND, reduced MCC; BHS may be the cause of symptoms such as frequency, urgency, and urge incontinence. It is common in various OAB and idiopathic hypersensitivity, which is characterized by reduced MCC and normal MABC; the latter includes psychogenic frequency syndrome. (2) Reduced bladder sensation: refers to delayed FD and ND, but SD and symptoms such as frequent voiding or bladder pain will not appear. It is common in diseases such as diabetic bladder dysfunction, sacral spinal cord NB, and chronic urinary retention caused by BOO. (3) Lack of bladder sensation: refers to patients who have completely lost bladder sensation, commonly seen in acute spinal cord lesions, sensory paralytic neuropathy, and other patients.

Detrusor Activity

Normal: The detrusor is stable during the bladder filling process, there is no uninhibited detrusor contraction, and it can inhibit the detrusor contraction induced by the irritation test.

Overactive detrusor: refers to the spontaneous or induced uninhibited contraction of the detrusor observed during the filling phase of UDS. It includes two modes: (1) phase-related overactive detrusor refers to the waveform changes that appear on the detrusor pressure curve during the bladder filling process, which may or may not cause urinary incontinence; (2) terminal overactive detrusor refers to the single, uninhibited detrusor contraction that occurs at the maximum bladder pressure volume on the detrusor pressure curve during the bladder filling, which cannot be inhibited and often leads to complete bladder emptying urinary incontinence.

Low detrusor activity: refers to the lack of contraction or low contraction force of the detrusor during the filling phase, often occurring in the bladder after obstruction, with the risk of overfilling the bladder.

Bladder Compliance

Normal bladder compliance: In a normal bladder, the detrusor pressure only experiences small changes (10–15 cmH_2O) from empty to full. If a normal bladder experiences a volume change of 400 mL from empty to full, its pressure change should be less than 10 cmH_2O, so the normal bladder compliance should be around 40 mL/cmH_2O; both too high and too low are abnormal.

Low bladder compliance: Many diseases can affect BC, and changes in BC are also the cause of LUTS. Low bladder compliance can be determined by three indicators: (1) a small change in bladder capacity is accompanied by a significant increase in bladder pressure; (2) bladder compliance value is less than 10 mL/cmH_2O; (3) end-of-fill pressure is greater than 15 cmH_2O. However, if the water injection speed is too fast, it can artificially cause a low compliance bladder, creating an illusion. To distinguish, you can stop injecting water. If the pressure drops, it is an illusion. If the pressure does not change, it is a low compliance bladder. The appearance of a low compliance bladder indicates an increase in collagen fibers in the bladder wall or a decrease in elastic fibers, reducing the viscoelastic function of the detrusor. This can be caused by BOO, local stimulation, long-term indwelling catheter, urinary diversion, bladder tuberculosis, or NB.

High bladder compliance: If the bladder capacity is more than twice the predicted bladder capacity and the pressure in the bladder is always low, it is called a high bladder compliance. Compared with a bladder without contraction, the detrusor of a high bladder compliance can contract, while the latter has no contraction. This can be caused by diabetes, complications of malignant anemia, spinal shock from spinal cord injury, sensory nerve damage, or repeated delayed voiding.

Bladder Capacity

Bladder capacity usually refers to functional bladder capacity, which is the maximum capacity of the bladder during the CMG process, which is the sum of the amount of urine expelled and the PVR. Less than 65% of the bladder capacity measurement suggests a small bladder capacity, while more than 150% of the bladder capacity measurement suggests a large bladder capacity. A small maximum bladder capacity can suggest a highly sensitive bladder (must be distinguished from sensory urgency), commonly seen in patients with interstitial cystitis, female idiopathic frequency syndrome, etc., with good compliance and stable detrusor muscle, and can also initiate voiding at will; pressure flow measurement shows no BOO.

Bladder safe capacity: The bladder safe capacity is the bladder capacity when the pressure in the bladder is less than 40 cmH_2O. When the pressure in the bladder exceeds the safe pressure, it can cause VUR, leading to upper urinary tract infection, kidney damage, and even kidney failure. Therefore, before CIC, use UDS to determine the bladder's safe capacity, and set the specific time point for CIC based on this, which is more in line with the physiological voiding of the bladder and more conducive to the recovery of bladder function.

Measurement of bladder safe capacity: UDS equipment can accurately measure the bladder safe capacity, but some patients have difficulty moving, and some hospitals lack urodynamic testing equipment, which makes it difficult to carry out. We can determine the patient's bladder safe capacity through a simple bladder pressure measurement technology.

Simple bladder pressure measurement (Fig. 12.1): Hang a 100 cm pressure ruler on the side of the infusion stand, a 500 mL saline bottle (with scale) at room temperature or heated to 35~37 °C. Connect a disposable bladder irrigator, expel the air, and hang it on the other side of the infusion stand; instruct the patient to empty the bladder as much as possible, assume a supine or sitting position, insert a sterile catheter, empty the urine in the bladder, and secure the catheter; connect one end of the bladder irrigator to the catheter and the other end to a sterile single-hole nasal oxygen tube, ensuring all tubes are connected smoothly; affix the graduated scale to the infusion stand, with the nasal oxygen tube closely aligned with the pressure scale; mark the zero point on the nasal oxygen tube at the same level as the patient's

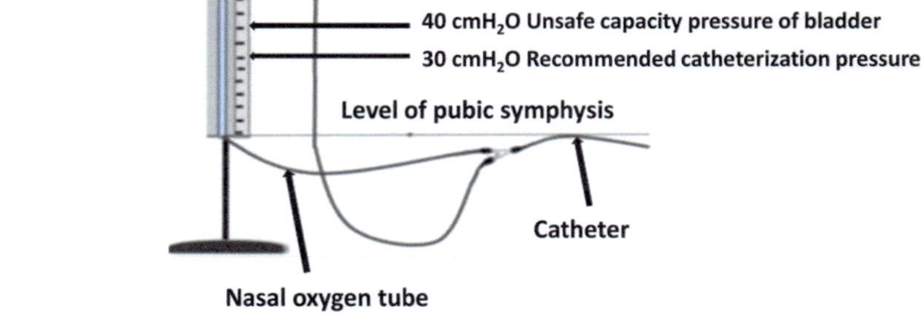

Fig. 12.1 Simple bladder pressure measurement method (you can also directly connect the catheter to a simple water column pressure gauge to determine if the bladder pressure during catheterization is safe)

pubic symphysis; open the infusion regulator to infuse saline into the bladder at an appropriate rate; observe the fluctuation of the water column in the pressure tube (expressed in cmH_2O to indicate pressure changes) for every certain volume entered; record the corresponding pressure changes with volume changes and the patient's own urge to urinate; when the water column in the pressure tube rises to 40 cmH_2O or above, stop the measurement when there is leakage at the urethral orifice; remove the measurement device, drain the bladder, remove the catheter, record the catheterization volume, and analyze it. You can also directly connect the catheter to a simple water column pressure gauge to determine if the bladder pressure at the time of catheterization is safe.

According to the simple bladder pressure measurement method, when the pressure reaches 40 cmH_2O, the amount of fluid drained is the safe bladder capacity; the safe bladder capacity includes the amount of sodium chloride injected plus the amount of urine generated in the bladder after catheterization; if the injection volume is >500 mL and the pressure is <40 cmH_2O, it is considered a "large bladder"; if the pressure reaches or is <40 cmH_2O and the injection volume is <300 mL, it is considered a "small bladder"; if the pressure reaches 40 cmH_2O when the injection volume is between 300 and 500 mL, it is considered a normal bladder capacity. By determining the patient's safe bladder capacity through simple bladder pressure measurement technology and determining the CIC time and frequency based on the safe bladder capacity, the patient's quality of life can be significantly improved.

Due to the guiding significance of safe bladder capacity for CIC, the simple bladder pressure measurement technology can only roughly reflect the bladder pressure and safe capacity rather than the detrusor pressure, so regular urodynamic examinations are still necessary to be performed for patients with long-term intermittent catheterization and conditions.

Detrusor Leak Point Pressure

During the bladder filling process, the pressure in bladder increases with the increase of the filling volume. When the pressure in the bladder exceeds the urethral pressure or urethral resistance, urine leakage occurs. At this point, the recorded detrusor pressure is the Detrusor Leak Point Pressure (DLPP).

DLPP measurement is a passive method of testing bladder storage pressure, bladder outlet resistance, and bladder compliance, effectively predicting the risk of upper urinary tract damage in patients with NB. A reference value of 40 cmH_2O is used for DLPP, with pressures >40 cmH_2O indicating a high risk of kidney damage. A higher DLPP implies a higher bladder pressure during storage, which can eventually lead to damage to the upper urinary tract over time. There is a close relationship between higher bladder pressure during storage, hydronephrosis, and kidney damage.

12.2.2.4 Pressure-Flow Measurement

Pressure-flow study (PFS) includes simultaneous recording of bladder pressure and urine flow rate. The function of the bladder and urethra is judged by analyzing the relationship between bladder pressure and various parameters of urine flow. In the early days of urodynamic research, the relationship between flow rate and voiding pressure was represented by the urethral resistance coefficient. The concept of the urethral resistance coefficient originates from the fluid mechanics of rigid pipes. The urethra is different from a rigid pipe because it is an irregular and expandable pipe. The urethral wall and surrounding tissues have active or passive activities, which can affect the passing urine flow. Therefore, the urethral resistance coefficient cannot be used as a parameter for effective comparison between different patients. The BOO defined by the ICS terminology and PFS can be anatomical or functional. Anatomical obstruction is due to the inability of the urethra to expand during voiding due to a narrow lumen, despite the relaxation of the urethral sphincter, the urine flow curve is still a continuous low flat curve. Functional urethral stenosis is when the urethral sphincter is in a contracted state during voiding, causing the urethra to narrow, which can be intermittent or continuous urethral contraction. Therefore, to distinguish between anatomical or functional urethral stenosis, urethral pressure or external urethral sphincter electromyogram should be recorded at the same time. Pressure recording usually includes bladder pressure measurement and abdominal pressure measurement, and the sphincter electromyogram (EMG) can also be recorded at the same time; the detrusor pressure is automatically calculated by the instrument pressure difference, that is, the value obtained after subtracting the abdominal pressure from the bladder pressure. This method can understand the information about the function of the detrusor and the urethra during voiding, and if the sphincter EMG is added, the coordination between the function of the detrusor and the activity of the sphincter can also be evaluated.

PFS can provide a detailed evaluation of voiding dysfunction, diagnose BOO, impaired detrusor contraction, and various NB dysfunctions.

12.2.3 Bladder Safety Pressure Measurement

Normally, the bladder pressure at the end of storage is 10–15 cmH_2O. When the bladder pressure during storage continuously exceeds 40 cmH_2O, the risk of bladder ureteral reflux and hydronephrosis significantly increases. Bladder ureteral reflux can significantly increase the risk of upper urinary tract infection and kidney damage caused by CIC. Therefore, bladder pressure is considered safe when it is ≤40 cmH_2O, and dangerous when it exceeds 40 cmH_2O.

Patients undergoing CIC should catheterize before the intravesical pressure reaches the safe bladder pressure to prevent urine reflux and protect the upper urinary tract function. It is recommended to perform CIC before the bladder volume reaches the dangerous volume or dangerous pressure. However, it is difficult to control the intravesical pressure to reach the safe bladder pressure during the normal procedure process, so we recommend catheterizing when the intravesical pressure of the patient reaches 30 cmH_2O (Fig. 12.2). At this time, catheterization can prevent excessive bladder pressure, reduce the risk of bladder ureter reflux, reduce unnecessary catheterization, reduce the risk of lower urinary tract injury, and improve the compliance of CIC patients. The bladder volume when the bladder pressure reaches 30 cmH_2O can be recorded through simple bladder pressure measurement or UDS, and then the bladder volume meter can be used to guide CIC. The voiding (catheterization) diary and bladder pressure volume measurement

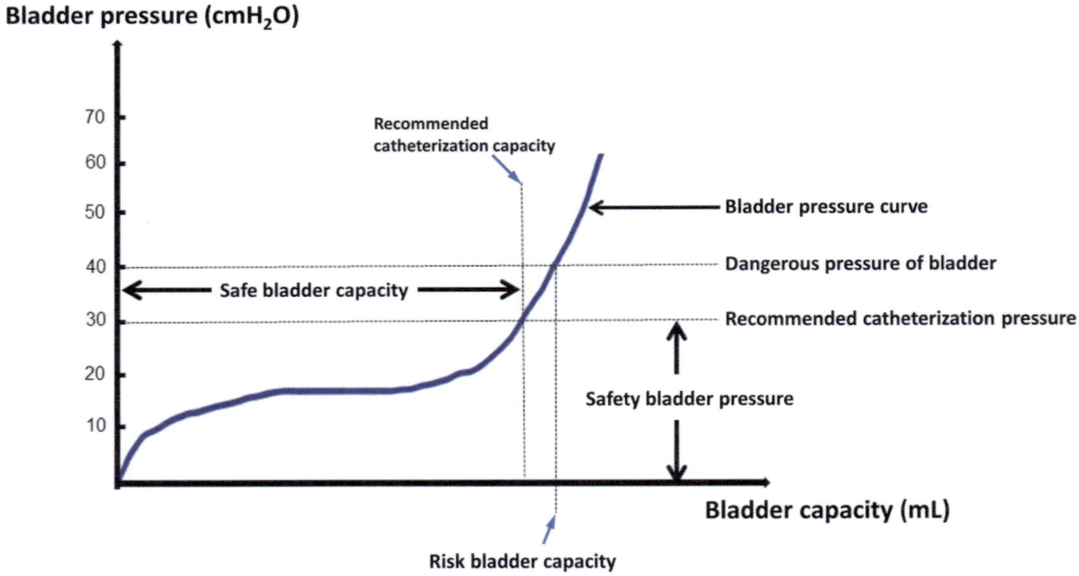

Fig. 12.2 Schematic of safe bladder pressure and safe volume

can help determine the safe bladder volume and safe pressure.

12.2.4 Voiding and Catheterization Diary

Most patients with NB have voiding disorders, including difficulty urinating and urinary incontinence [19]. Recording a catheterization diary or voiding + catheterization diary can understand the single voided volume, the number of incontinence occurrences, and the amount of leakage. For patients undergoing CIC treatment, the volume of each catheterization and the time of catheterization can be recorded, providing a basis for the adjustment of the subsequent treatment plan [20].

12.2.5 Questionnaire Survey

Conduct a questionnaire survey on patients to understand the effect evaluation and quality of life improvement of patients after CIC treatment, and guide patients' CIC based on the survey results.

12.2.5.1 CIC Difficulty Questionnaire (ICDQ) [21] (Table 12.1)

This questionnaire includes 13 specific indicators such as pain, resistance, bleeding, and leakage during the catheterization process, making the inquiry process more comprehensive and quantifying the difficulty of the catheterization process. These symptoms may indicate spasms of the urethral sphincter, urethral stenosis, and perforation. A study of 70 patients with urinary retention undergoing long-term CIC showed that the average ICDQ scores for catheterization due to different primary diseases were quite different. Among them, the average ICDQ score for patients with spinal cord injury undergoing CIC was the lowest, at 0.7 points.

12.2.5.2 Intermittent Catheterization Satisfaction Questionnaire (InCaSaQ) [22] (Table 12.2)

InCaSaQ quantifies satisfaction and provides an effective tool for evaluating patients' satisfaction with CIC. A large sample survey showed that the average InCaSaQ score of CIC patients was 2.3 points (2 points for satisfaction and 3 points for very satisfaction).

12.2.5.3 Patient Quality of Life Score (SF-36 Score)

In-depth inquiry into the various issues mentioned in the SF-36 questionnaire can assess the patient's physical and mental health and the impact and limitations of CIC on daily activities [23].

Close follow-up and comprehensive guidance for patients undergoing CIC are important measures to improve CIC compliance and reduce the difficulty and discomfort of catheterization.

Table 12.1 Intermittent Catheterization Difficulty Questionnaire (ICDQ) frequency and intensity during the CIC process

The process of CIC	Frequency				Discomfort intensity			
	Never–0	Occasionally–1	Often–2	Always–3	None–0	A little–1	Often–2	Always–3
CIC brought me discomfort. I encountered less resistance. I didn't have to insert the catheter or wait								
I encountered resistance and had to wait a while before I could continue to insert the catheter								
I encountered resistance and needed to push hard to continue to insert the catheter								
There is always resistance in the process of catheter insertion								
There is serious resistance during insertion. I need to pause CIC. I need to change my position or use my hand to help reduce resistance before I can continue to insert								
I have leg spasms, leg pain, chills, headache, sweating, and other symptoms								
I have urethral bleeding								

(continued)

Table 12.1 (continued)

The process of CIC	Frequency				Discomfort intensity			
	Never–0	Occasionally–1	Often–2	Always–3	None–0	A little–1	Often–2	Always–3
I need to change my position to empty my bladder								
There is a sense of resistance when pulling out the catheter								
Urinary incontinence occurred during CIC								
There will be pain after catheterization								

Table 12.2 Intermittent Catheterization Satisfaction Questionnaire (InCaSaQ)

Question		Not satisfied	Lightly satisfied	Satisfied	Very satisfied
Packing	About the fineness and volume of packaging				
	About the hygiene and firmness of packaging				
	On the opening and fixation of catheters				
Lubrication	About the way of lubrication used				
Mode	Self-lubrication, gel lubrication, water lubrication				
Catheter	On the question of holding, pushing, and inserting the urethra				
	About the ease and comfort of insertion				
	On the convenience of urination (length of catheter and catheter attachment)				
After catheterization	On whether it is convenient to handle the catheter after use				

References

1. Vahter L, Zopp I, Kreegipuu M, et al. Clean intermittent self-catheterization in persons with multiple sclerosis: the influence of cognitive dysfunction [J]. Mult Scler. 2009;15(3):379–84. https://doi.org/10.1177/1352458508098599.
2. Wilson M. Clean intermittent self-catheterisation: working with patients [J]. Br J Nurs. 2015;24(2):76, 78, 80 passim. https://doi.org/10.12968/bjon.2015.24.2.76.
3. Liao L. Evaluation and management of neurogenic bladder: what is new in China? [J]. Int J Mol Sci. 2015;16(8):18580–600.
4. Vainrib M, Stav K, Gruenwald I, et al. [Position statement for intermittent catheterization of urinary bladder] [J]. Harefuah. 2018;157(4):257–61.
5. Okamoto I, Prieto J, Avery M, et al. Intermittent catheter users' symptom identification, description and management of urinary tract infection: a qualitative study [J]. BMJ Open. 2017;7(9):e016453. https://doi.org/10.1136/bmjopen-2017-016453.

6. Lotfinejad N, Peters A, Tartari E, et al. Hand hygiene in health care: 20 years of ongoing advances and perspectives [J]. Lancet Infect Dis. 2021;21(8):e209–21. https://doi.org/10.1016/s1473-3099(21)00383-2.
7. Bradley CS, Smith KE, Kreder KJ. Urodynamic evaluation of the bladder and pelvic floor [J]. Gastroenterol Clin N Am. 2008;37(3):539–52, vii. https://doi.org/10.1016/j.gtc.2008.06.006.
8. Amarenco G, Sheikh Ismaël S, Chesnel C, et al. Diagnosis and clinical evaluation of neurogenic bladder [J]. Eur J Phys Rehabil Med. 2017;53(6):975–80. https://doi.org/10.23736/s1973-9087.17.04992-9.
9. Laquerre J. Hydronephrosis: diagnosis, grading, and treatment [J]. Radiol Technol. 2020;92(2):135–51.
10. Yadav P, Alsabban A, De Los Reyes T, et al. A systematic review of paediatric neurogenic lower urinary tract dysfunction guidelines using the Appraisal of Guidelines and Research Evaluation (AGREE) II instrument [J]. BJU Int. 2023;131(5):520–9. https://doi.org/10.1111/bju.15902.
11. Mallya A, Karthikeyan VS, Manohar CMS, Keshavamurthy R. Bilateral retrograde pyelography leading to anuria [J]. Natl Med J India. 2019;32(1):20–1. https://doi.org/10.4103/0970-258x.272110.
12. Lúcio A, Lourenço CB, Damasceno BP, et al. The effect of pelvic floor muscle contraction on detrusor overactivity pressure in neurogenic and nonneurogenic women during urodynamic study: a cross-sectional study [J]. Am J Phys Med Rehabil. 2019;98(4):275–9. https://doi.org/10.1097/phm.0000000000001065.
13. Ansari SH, Mahdy AE. Are video-urodynamics superior to traditional urodynamic studies in changing treatment decision with urinary symptoms? [J]. Arab J Urol. 2019;17(2):160–5. https://doi.org/10.1080/2090598x.2019.1590518.
14. Rosier P, Schaefer W, Lose G, et al. International Continence Society Good Urodynamic Practices and Terms 2016: urodynamics, uroflowmetry, cystometry, and pressure-flow study [J]. Neurourol Urodyn. 2017;36(5):1243–60. https://doi.org/10.1002/nau.23124.
15. Dolgun NZ, Jones K, Harmanli O. Voided volume for postoperative voiding assessment following prolapse and urinary incontinence surgery [J]. Int Urogynecol J. 2021;32(3):587–91. https://doi.org/10.1007/s00192-020-04346-w.
16. Kato S, Watanabe H, Yamasue K. Freeflow: the novel portable uroflowmeter can help to realize practical urinary conditions at home [J]. Low Urin Tract Symptoms. 2022;14(3):208–13. https://doi.org/10.1111/luts.12426.
17. Serlin DC, Heidelbaugh JJ, Stoffel JT. Urinary retention in adults: evaluation and initial management [J]. Am Fam Physician. 2018;98(8):496–503.
18. Seth JH, Panicker JN, Fowler CJ. The neurological organization of micturition [J]. Handb Clin Neurol. 2013;117:111–7. https://doi.org/10.1016/b978-0-444-53491-0.00010-9.
19. Bright E, Cotterill N, Drake M, Abrams P. Developing a validated urinary diary: phase 1 [J]. Neurourol Urodyn. 2012;31(5):625–33.
20. Bright E, Drake MJ, Abrams P. Urinary diaries: evidence for the development and validation of diary content, format, and duration [J]. Neurourol Urodyn. 2011;30(3):348–52. https://doi.org/10.1002/nau.20994.
21. Zachariou A, Zachariou D, Kaltsas A, et al. Translation and validation of the Intermittent Catheterization Difficulty Questionnaire (ICDQ) into Greek [J]. J Multidiscip Healthc. 2022;15:2571–7.
22. Guinet-Lacoste A, Jousse M, Verollet D, et al. Validation of the InCaSaQ, a new tool for the evaluation of patient satisfaction with clean intermittent self-catheterization [J]. Ann Phys Rehabil Med. 2014;57(3):159–68.
23. Fumincelli L, Mazzo A, Martins JCA, et al. Quality of life of intermittent urinary catheterization users and their caregivers: a scoping review [J]. Worldviews Evid-Based Nurs. 2017;14(4):324–33. https://doi.org/10.1111/wvn.12231.

Focus on the Treatment and Prevention of CIC Complications

13

Jian-Guo Wen

CIC is an effective method to ensure bladder emptying, but there is a 2–8% complication rate during its application, especially prevalent in patients who perform CIC for a long time. The most common complications are urinary tract infection (UTI), followed by complications related to the urethra, testicles, epididymis and bladder. To ensure the smooth progress of CIC, it is very important to focus on the treatment and prevention of CIC complications [1].

13.1 Urinary Tract Infection

UTI induced by CIC belongs to the category of catheter-associated urinary tract infection (CAUTI), which is the most common complication of CIC. Compared with the general population, patients who perform CIC have a higher risk of UTI and kidney deterioration. When urethral injury or bladder wall injury occurs, the mucosal barrier is damaged and infected. The bladder wall is easily invaded by bacteria in the PVR. When the bladder is filled with PVR, capillaries are blocked, preventing the transmission of metabolic and immune substrates to the bladder wall [2].

J.-G. Wen (✉)
Pediatric Urodynamic Center/Department of Urology, First Affiliated Hospital of Zhengzhou University, Zhengzhou, China

Due to significant differences in the definition and reporting methods of UTI, it is difficult to determine its true incidence, prevalence, and relative risk. UTI, as a complication of CIC, has been reported at an incidence rate of about 2.5 times per person per year, and more than 80% of patients have experienced at least one UTI within 5 years. The incidence of CAUTI combined with pyelonephritis is about 5%. It has not been able to determine the incidence of CAUTI between various CIC techniques (such as single-use and multiple-use, clean, and sterile catheterization), which may be due to an unreasonable research design or a small number of patients. EAU's guidelines on neurogenic bladder dysfunction suggest that sterile CIC is the most appropriate option when considering the incidence of UTI. Aseptic technology is defined as "keeping the catheter sterile, disinfecting the genitalia, and using disinfectant lubricants" [3].

13.1.1 Causes of CAUTI

13.1.1.1 Incorrect Catheterization Technique

The reasons for UTI due to catheterization technique include (1) insufficient number of catheterizations; (2) insufficient urine drainage during catheterization; (3) poor catheterization technique and improper catheter care; (4) insufficient fluid intake; (5) excessive intake of liquid food;

J.-G. Wen (ed.), *Progress in Clean Intermittent Catheterization*, Experts' Perspectives on Medical Advances, https://doi.org/10.1007/978-981-97-5021-4_13

(6) and catheterization injury. For details on CIC-related UTI and its treatment measures, see Table 13.1.

CAUTI may be caused by poor catheterization technique or contamination before the catheter reaches the bladder, or it may be caused by the formation of biofilms (microorganisms that settle on the inner surface of the catheter). Under unfavorable conditions (repeated use of the catheter), the organisms will detach from the biofilm and float freely in the urine, which may lead to symptomatic infection.

Currently, there is no clear research showing that changing catheter insertion techniques, catheter types, or catheterization strategies can improve the incidence of urinary tract infections [4]. Recurrent symptomatic UTI is a problem for many patients undergoing long-term CIC.

Treatment should be considered if a clinical infection occurs [5].

13.1.1.2 Gender Factors

Amongst patients undergoing CIC, UTI is more likely to occur in women. Woodbury, Hayes, and Askes reported that in a community, 912 spinal cord injury patients needed to undergo CIC, half of whom were women [6]. The number of urinary tract infections in women was significantly higher than in men. Factors related to urinary tract infections include a higher average number of catheter insertions, CIC performed by caregivers, etc. Moy and Wein reported that the longer the catheterization time, the higher the incidence of UTI; paraplegic patients who rely on wheelchairs often enter heavily contaminated public toilets for CIC, and neglect of basic

Table 13.1 CIC-related UTI and its treatment measures

Cause	Mechanism	Measures
Insufficient emptying frequency	Insufficient emptying frequency can lead to excessive bladder capacity and prolonged urine retention time, increasing the risk of urinary tract infection	Regular CIC can prevent bacteria from migrating into the bladder, thus causing symptomatic infection
Insufficient emptying during catheterization	The residual amount left in the bladder after catheterization promotes bacterial proliferation	Ensure bladder emptying; the patient should perform gentle Credé maneuver when removing the catheter
Insufficient fluid intake	Insufficient fluid intake. When producing low urine volume (less than 1200 mL/day), patients tend to reduce the number of catheterizations, and the urine stagnation time is prolonged	Total daily fluid intake (from food and all types of beverages) is about 2.7 L/day for adult women and about 3.7 L/day for adult men
Poor catheterization technique and inadequate catheter care	Poor catheterization technique and inadequate catheter care introduce bacteria into the bladder	Reassess the catheterization technique of the person inserting the catheter. Consider the use of sterile catheters
Excessive fluid intake	Excessive fluid intake leads to an increase in urine volume; if the number of catheterizations cannot be adjusted or is not adjusted in time, it leads to high bladder pressure and risk of bladder overdistension	Adjust fluid intake or adjust the frequency of CIC. Small amounts of fluid every hour between breakfast and dinner; then reduce intake
Nocturia	Some patients (such as those with spinal cord injuries and/or multiple sclerosis and older patients) may have nocturia, which is related to insufficient secretion of nocturnal antidiuretic hormone or kidney dilation or impaired heart condition	Avoid consuming large amounts of fluid at night. Increase the frequency of CIC at night Take desmopressin before sleep; monitor serum sodium levels
Catheterization injury	The damage to the bladder, urothelial, and urethral mucosa during catheterization increases the risk of infection	Evaluate catheterization techniques to help correct incorrect insertion techniques. Consider another type of catheter material (Coudé tip, hydrophilic coating) to facilitate passage. Consult a urologist

hygiene prevention techniques may be more likely to cause UTI [7, 8].

13.1.2 CAUTI Diagnosis

1. Urine analysis. There are usually four methods available for diagnosing UTI. (1) More than five white blood cells in the urine sediment per high power field, UTI should be suspected. (2) Bacteria found in unstained urine sediment per high power field. (3) Urine leukocyte esterase test can reflect the enzyme produced by the decomposition of white blood cells in urine. (4) Nitrite test in urine, ingested nitrate will be decomposed into nitrite by gram-positive bacteria in urine, so nitrite in urine can be detected to diagnose UTI. Currently, one or several tests of urine analysis can replace urine culture; these tests can predict the positive results of urine culture.
2. Urine culture. It is the main method for diagnosing UTI. The bladder is normally sterile, but when urine is excreted, it can be contaminated with miscellaneous bacteria through the external urethral orifice. To reduce these influencing factors, clean midstream urine is often taken for urine culture. However, if children with NB have persistent abnormal voiding and it is inconvenient to retain clean midstream urine, a catheter can be used to obtain urine specimens. The cleanliness of the vulva before catheterization and the cleanliness procedure during catheterization are crucial. In addition, bacterial colony counts need to be done for growing bacteria at urine culture. If the number of bacteria in the clean midstream urine culture is $>10^8$/L, it can be diagnosed. If it is between 10^7/L and 10^8/L, it is suspicious, and if it is $<10^7$/L, it is considered contamination. If the number of bacteria in the catheter specimen reaches 10^7/L, infection should be considered. If bacteria grow in the urine sample taken through bladder puncture, UTI should be diagnosed.
3. The diagnosis of CAUTI should include the presence of clinical symptoms of UTI and meeting the UTI diagnostic criteria, namely, the number of white blood cells in the centrifugal sediment of clean midstream urine routine is $\geq$5/high power field (HP). The number of bacteria in the clean midstream urine culture is $>10^8$/L, and the number of bacteria in the catheter specimen is $\geq10^7$/L.

13.1.3 Types and Treatment of UTI in CIC

1. Common types of UTI include bacteriuria and pyuria. Bacteriuria refers to the presence of a large number of bacteria in the urine, including pseudobacteriuria and true bacteriuria. True bacteriuria refers to those who have positive bacterial culture of bladder puncture urine or those who have $\geq10^5$ CFU/mL bacterial colonies in the morning midstream urine culture, and if the bacteria are the same, it can be diagnosed. If true bacteriuria is present, it can be diagnosed as urinary tract infection. Pyuria refers to the presence of a large number of white blood cells in the urine caused by urinary tract infection causing mucosal damage and a large number of inflammatory cells infiltrating.
2. Treatment principles: In patients undergoing CIC treatment, only symptomatic UTI needs to be treated. Treatment measures include retaining the catheter (or cystostomy) for continuous urine drainage and using antibiotics, etc. The choice and duration of antibiotics will be carried out in accordance with the relevant provisions of rational use of antibiotics.

13.1.4 Prevention of UTI

Literature reports that the main risk factors for urinary tract infection caused by CIC include improper catheterization technique, insufficient fluid intake, low catheterization frequency, and inadequate training (education), while secondary factors include overfilled bladder, being female, non-hydrophilic catheter, etc. Therefore, to prevent UTI, the following steps should be focused.

1. Strengthen training and education. Currently, there is a lack of educational materials on CIC in China, so it is required that health-care workers explain thoroughly to patients, not only fully addressing their doubts but also fully comforting their emotions, letting patients accept CIC from their hearts, and carrying out CIC in a relaxed and standard manner.
2. Adhering to basic daily preventive habits may help avoid urinary tract infections in high-risk CIC populations, for example, maintaining hand and perineal hygiene.
3. Strictly catheterize according to the number of times recommended by the specialist. Fewer catheterizations will lead to a higher urinary volume of catheterization and increase the risk of urinary system infections in patients. Therefore, a reasonable number of catheterizations and avoiding overfilling of the bladder are extremely important preventive measures. For most adults, perform catheterization four to six times a day. If the number of catheterizations is too high, it will increase the chance of introducing harmful bacteria, thereby increasing the occurrence of infections [9].
4. Dietary adjustment. One measure that may reduce infections is to consume cranberry juice, foods containing lactic acid bacteria, and vitamin C [10]. Preliminary research confirms that cranberries can inhibit *E. coli* from adhering to the urinary epithelial wall [11]. In a community-based survey, Woodbury and others surveyed spinal cord injury patients in CIC and found that those who took cranberry or vitamin C supplements reduced the incidence of UTI. Hess and his colleagues conducted a small, randomized, double-blind, placebo-controlled study, compared with the control group, and found that the risk of urinary tract infection in the group taking cranberry tablets has been reduced.
5. Choose the right catheter. In recent years, a large number of clinical studies including randomized controlled trials have shown that the use of hydrophilic coated catheters can reduce the occurrence of urinary tract infections. Cardenas and others conducted a clinical experimental study on 224 acute traumatic spinal cord injury patients in 15 spinal cord injury centers in North America, and it showed that the first time symptomatic urinary system infection requiring antibiotic treatment was significantly delayed in patients using hydrophilic-coated catheters for CIC compared to patients using uncoated regular PVC catheters (with lubricating oil). At the same time, it reduced the incidence of urinary tract infections during hospitalization by 21%. Compared to regular catheters, hydrophilic catheters can reduce the friction between the ureter and the urethra, thereby minimizing the minor trauma caused by catheterization and reducing the occurrence of urinary system infections. Moreover, the overall satisfaction rate of hydrophilic catheters in terms of convenience and comfort is relatively high, making patients more willing to accept and use them long term. A randomized trial study on healthy male volunteers also yielded the same results [12].
6. Common preventive measures for CIC-related UTIs
   (a) Maintain hygiene, especially of the hands and perineum: Hands should be thoroughly washed before catheterization. The genitals should be cleaned daily with soap and water, always washing from front to back. It is best to catheterize before defecation to minimize contamination of the urethra by *E. coli*. It is recommended to clean the perineum immediately after sexual intercourse, as intercourse may push anal bacteria into the urethra. In sexually active women, avoid using spermicidal lubricants, as these products may alter the normal vaginal and lower urinary tract flora.
   (b) Instruct male patients to correctly position the male urethra during the catheter insertion process to minimize trauma caused by the catheter passing through the curved part of the urethra.

(c) Be careful to avoid touching the tip of the catheter and/or allowing it to touch other surfaces.
(d) If postmenopausal female patients have insufficient estrogen in the perineal tissue, consider using vaginal estrogen medication.
(e) Use a large amount of lubricant along the catheter (especially for male patients), as a dry catheter may cause an increase in urethral secretions, leading to bacterial contamination.
(f) Encourage patients to catheterize at least four to six times a day to empty the bladder as much as possible. Prevent overfilling of the bladder.
(g) Encourage the use of a new catheter each time CIC is performed. Most catheters are manufactured and packaged for sterile use only.
(h) Acidification of the bladder may prevent bacterial growth. In populations without catheter treatment, cranberries have been suggested to prevent the growth of intestinal bacteria in the urethra and bladder. Some patients may be restricted from taking cranberries (such as those prone to producing oxalates or uric acid). Anticoagulant therapy patients are not allowed to use cranberries, and it is not recommended for this population. *Lactobacillus* in the diet (yogurt) has been proven to prevent the growth of *E. coli* in the urethra.

13.1.5 CAUTI Treatment and Prevention [13]

13.1.5.1 Drug Treatment

Rapid diagnosis of CAUTI and rational use of antibiotics are keys to effectively controlling infection and preventing upper urinary tract damage. During the acute phase of CAUTI, urine should be collected correctly for quantitative bacterial culture as soon as possible before applying antibiotics. Clinically, before the drug sensitivity results are obtained, using antibiotics based on experience is often required, and rapid use of potent antibiotics can prevent the formation of renal scars. The mechanisms of action of different antimicrobial drugs vary, mainly divided into the following types: (1) inhibiting the synthesis of the pathogen's cell wall, promoting the pathogen to swell and rupture in a hypotonic environment; (2) inhibiting protein synthesis; (3) increasing the permeability of the pathogen's cell membrane, causing the pathogen to die from imbalance. Therefore, it is necessary to choose the appropriate type of antibiotic according to the pathogen. Misuse of antibiotics not only makes it difficult to achieve therapeutic effects and affects disease control but also enhances the resistance of pathogens.

After long-term and widespread use of penicillins, pathogens generally have high resistance. Among them, the resistance rate of *E. coli* producing ESBL to amoxicillin has exceeded 88%, and the resistance rate to meropenem and ampicillin is also high. However, amoxicillin and ampicillin still have high antimicrobial activity against *Enterococcus faecalis* and can be selected for clinical treatment based on drug sensitivity tests. Piperacillin/tazobactam is a semi-synthetic penicillin drug, which is stable to β-lactamase and has certain antimicrobial activity against ESBL-producing strains. It can be used in the treatment of complex UTIs caused by ESBL-producing strains. The first- to third-generation cephalosporins are often used orally in the treatment of non-complex UTIs. With the long-term irrational use of cephalosporins, the spread of cephalosporin-resistant pathogens and the increase in ESBL-producing strains have occurred. Commonly used first- and second-generation cephalosporins such as cefuroxime have poor therapeutic effects in children with NB and UTI. The drug sensitivity of third-generation cephalosporins is also not optimistic, indicating that the resistance and multiple resistance phenomena caused by the widespread use of cephalosporins are becoming more serious. Some of the antibiotics selected in clinical practice include ceftriaxone, cefotiam, cefoperazone, etc., which should be used based on drug sensitivity [14].

Carbapenems are atypical β-lactam antibiotics with the broadest antimicrobial spectrum and the strongest antimicrobial activity and have become one of the main antimicrobial drugs for the treatment of severe bacterial infections. They mainly include meropenem, imipenem, and ertapenem. Carbapenems have certain antimicrobial activity against Gram-positive bacteria, Gram-negative bacteria, and anaerobic bacteria. Except for being hydrolyzed by carbapenemase, they are stable against other β-lactamases. These drugs are often used in the treatment of severe complex UTIs caused by ESBL-producing Gram-negative bacteria. Ertapenem has a longer half-life and can be administered once a day. It can treat community-acquired complex UTIs caused by ESBL-producing Gram-negative bacteria, but it cannot treat methicillin-resistant *Staphylococcus aureus* (MRSA) and vancomycin-resistant enterococci (VRE). Meropenem and imipenem can treat hospital-acquired Gram-positive and Gram-negative bacteria complex UTI, but they cannot treat MRSA and VRE infections. Doripenem belongs to a new type of drug, which has a better therapeutic effect on hospital-acquired complex UTI, has certain antibacterial activity against Gram-positive bacteria, but cannot treat MRSA and VRE infections [15]. It has better activity against some *Pseudomonas aeruginosa* infections than meropenem and should be reserved for patients with severe infections caused by *Pseudomonas aeruginosa*, multiple pathogens, and multidrug-resistant Gram-negative bacteria. After the widespread use of carbapenems, it can exacerbate the resistance and multidrug resistance of many types of pathogens. Some studies have pointed out that carbapenem-resistant pathogens have been reported in clinical practice, so their use should be strictly controlled [16].

Quinolone antibacterial drugs are artificially synthesized drugs that selectively inhibit bacterial DNA gyrase. Ciprofloxacin and levofloxacin have antibacterial activity against Gram-negative bacteria, but they are not strong against Gram-positive bacteria. Levofloxacin and ciprofloxacin are first-line treatment drugs for non-complex UTI, and they are more applicable in areas with high resistance rates to compound sulfamethoxazole. Some studies have pointed out that the resistance rates of *E. coli* producing ESBLs to ciprofloxacin and levofloxacin are both 86.3%, and *Klebsiella pneumoniae* producing ESBLs have resistance rates to the above two drugs of 46.2% and 50%. Quinolone drugs have a broad antibacterial spectrum and have special activity against *Pseudomonas aeruginosa*. They are widely used in adults, but they should be used with caution because they can affect the development of children's cartilage. Polymyxin antibacterial drugs are bacterial wall detergents, which can kill *Pseudomonas aeruginosa*, ESBLs-producing Gram-negative bacteria (except for Proteus), and have a good therapeutic effect on complex UTI caused by multidrug-resistant Gram-negative bacteria. Due to the increasing incidence of infections caused by multidrug-resistant Gram-negative bacteria and the lack of effective anti-*Pseudomonas* drugs, polymyxin drugs have begun to be re-applied to the treatment of complex UTI caused by multidrug-resistant bacteria. The commonly used preparations include colistin, polymyxin B, and colistimethate sodium, but renal toxicity reactions are prone to occur after medication, so children need to use them with caution. Amphotericin B, fluconazole, itraconazole, and other drugs are more common in drug resistance and are often not used alone.

Clinically, the first choice can be the enzyme inhibitor piperacillin tazobactam for anti-infection treatment. In children, the total daily intravenous dose is 30–100 mg/kg by weight, divided into three doses, that is, once every 8 hours; the course of treatment is at least 1 week; stop the medication when the routine urine test turns negative and the urine culture is negative twice. Continue to take orally amoxicillin, cephalosporins, or furazolidone enteric-coated tablets until the outpatient follow-up. For those with urinary culture pathogens indicating resistance to piperacillin tazobactam, choose antibiotics based on drug sensitivity tests. Carbapenem antibiotics have high sensitivity to pathogens and are generally used for severe infections. For children aged 3 months to 12 years, depending on the type of infection, severity, pathogen sensitivity, and specific patient conditions, meropenem is given every 8 hours at a dose of 10–20 mg/kg. Stop the medication when the routine urine test turns negative and the urine culture is negative twice. The efficacy and tolerance of this product in infants under 3 months are unclear. During the treatment of infection, if multiple pathogens are cultured in the urine, combined medication should be used according to the results of drug sensitivity. Some studies have pointed out that instilling gentamicin into the bladder can control infection and achieve good therapeutic effects.

NB patients' secondary reflux increases the risk of pyelonephritis. For patients with recurrent UTI accompanied by VUR, prophylactic antibiotics should be started after infection control to prevent inflammation from damaging the kidneys and to allow time for low-grade reflux to disappear naturally or for high-grade reflux surgery. The selected prophylactic antibiotics should have broad-spectrum antimicrobial activity, be inexpensive, have high concentrations in urine, and have low toxicity to children. The preventive dose should be 1/3 to 1/2 of the treatment dose, generally taken before bedtime to allow the drug to stay in the urine for a longer time. Clinically, prophylactic antibiotics can be chosen as furazolidone enteric-coated tablets or oral cephalosporins such as cefaclor and cefuroxime. For children over 1 month, the treatment dose of furazolidone enteric-coated tablets is 5–7 mg/kg per day according to body weight, and the preventive dose is 1/3 to 1/2 taken every night. The common dose of cefaclor for children is 20–40 mg/kg per day, divided into three doses (every 8 hours), and the preventive dose is 1/3 to 1/2 taken every night. Newborns should use this drug with caution.

13.1.5.2 Surgical Treatment

Small bladder capacity, persistent urinary bladder control dysfunction, VUR, etc. are important factors causing or leading to recurrent UTI. Surgery should be considered in the following situations: (1) obvious neurological lesions; (2) persistent shrinkage of bladder capacity; (3) drugs cannot control or prevent infection; (4) decline in kidney function; (5) significant inhibition of kidney growth; (6) progressive renal scarring, etc.

13.1.5.3 Supportive Treatment

Continue CIC under fully disinfected and clean conditions, appropriately rehydrate, and alkalinize urine.

In summary, UTI is one of the most common complications of CIC. Asymptomatic bacteriuria does not require treatment. However, those with fever or significant increase in urinary leukocytes need to collect urine for bacterial culture and apply antibiotic treatment. If necessary, stop CIC and switch to bladder fistula for urine drainage.

13.2 Urinary Tract-Related Complications [17]

13.2.1 Pain and Discomfort

Patients with intact urethral mucosa and nerves may experience pain and discomfort during the process of catheter insertion or removal, as well as when bladder spasms or urinary tract infections occur. Incomplete relaxation of pelvic floor muscles or mucosal atrophy in elderly women can cause pain during the process of catheter insertion or removal. During the CIC training period, fear of pain may affect learning and mental relaxation. Severe pain during catheter insertion significantly affects quality of life. Therefore, patients who are about to undergo CIC should be trained to help them master methods to alleviate pain as much as possible.

1. Prevention: Ask about the patient's medical history to understand the patient's urethral sensation. Many NB patients have dull or lost urethral sensation, so there is no problem of urethral pain during catheterization. But for other patients, urethral pain during CIC may be very significant. Whether CIC causes urethral pain varies greatly among individuals. For patients with sensitive urethra, the following measures can be taken for prevention: (1) Choose a smaller size catheter as much as possible. (2) Proper catheter lubrication and

correct urethral positioning can alleviate urethral pain, especially male urethral pain. (3) Use lidocaine cream on the catheter or local anesthetic ointment in the urethra before catheterization. In women, lack of estrogen in the urethra and perineal tissues may cause pain. Over time, the pain and discomfort during catheter insertion usually decrease.
2. Treatment: Generally, the pain subsides or disappears after the catheter is removed. A very small number of patients continue to feel pain in the short term, which can be relieved by oral analgesics. In addition, tension and anxiety are risk factors for discomfort and pain, so patients should be as relaxed as possible during the catheter insertion process.

13.2.2 Urethritis

Urethritis is one of the main complications during the CIC process in men. Historical studies have shown that the incidence of urethritis in patients undergoing CIC treatment is between 1% and 18%. It is often caused by too frequent catheterization and poor awareness of cleanliness. However, the material characteristics of the catheter and catheterization techniques have changed significantly in recent years, and it is obviously unscientific to directly apply historical experience to current patients. There is still a lack of data on the incidence of urethritis and related risk factors.

1. Prevention: The process of catheterization should be clean. Regularly drink water to avoid too frequent catheterization.
2. Treatment: Generally, no special treatment is required. If a urinary tract infection occurs, infection control treatment should be carried out.

13.2.3 Prostatitis

This situation often occurs in adult CIC, with the reported incidence rate being 18–31%.

1. Prevention: Strictly follow the CIC procedure to perform CIC.
2. Treatment: Patients who perform CIC and develop prostatitis should be treated with antibiotics. The treatment should follow a standardized plan, usually using antibiotics for 4 weeks, reaching a high concentration in the prostate, and performing suprapubic cystostomy during the acute phase.

13.2.4 Urethral Bleeding [18]

During the initial procedure of CIC, patients often experience urethral bleeding, which is manifested as blood at the top of the catheter after catheterization; occasionally the color of the urine is red; this situation is not a big problem. It is reported that one-third of patients who need long-term CIC will regularly experience urethral bleeding. Persistent urethral bleeding in patients with long-term CIC may be a sign of UTI.

1. Prevention: The catheterization movement should be gentle. In males, the three bends of the urethra should be handled correctly. If the resistance is high when inserting the catheter, stop immediately for 3–5 seconds. Females can slightly rotate the catheter and then continue, but do not force it in.
2. Treatment: This symptom generally disappears after 1 week, some may last for 2 weeks, and this generally does not require treatment. If persistent urethral bleeding occurs, a routine urine test and urine culture should be performed to determine whether there is a urinary tract infection. If there is, treat it according to the urinary tract infection, and normal clean CIC can be performed during this period. If there is no urinary tract infection or the treatment effect of urinary tract infection is not good, stop clean CIC temporarily, try again after 3–5 days, abdominal pressure voiding or indwelling catheter can be used during this period, and this situation is very rare.

13.2.5 Formation of False Passage [19]

The formation of a urethral false passage is a common complication of CIC, often seen in patients with urethral stricture or enlarged prostate. The false passage may occur at the location of the external sphincter of the urethra, which is the distal end of the prostate. Patients with urethral stricture, detrusor-sphincter dyssynergia, and enlarged prostate should be alert to the formation of a urethral false passage.

1. Prevention: Familiarize with the patient's urethral anatomy to avoid violent catheterization. Attention should be paid to patients with urethral stricture or enlarged prostate.
2. Treatment: Urethral injury during CIC can lead to the formation of false passages, with the catheter entering the false passage instead of the bladder, making it impossible to complete CIC treatment. In this case, antibiotics should be used, and the catheter should be retained for continuous drainage for 2–3 weeks.

13.2.6 Urethral Injury

Urethral injury is common in patients undergoing CIC, especially in the early stages, with up to 30% of patients experiencing urethral bleeding. Insufficient lubrication or overly violent insertion of the catheter can cause urethral spasms, which, if not adjusted in time, can lead to urethral injury, causing both urethral bleeding and the formation of false passages.

1. Prevention: Fully lubricate the catheter before catheterization; if there is significant resistance during insertion, stop immediately for 3–5 seconds. Women can slightly rotate the catheter and then continue; avoid violent catheterization to prevent urethral spasms.
2. Treatment: In patients with neurogenic dysfunction, the use of hydrophilic-coated catheters can significantly reduce the incidence of microscopic hematuria. Using lubricants can reduce the risk of urethral injury. Adjust the catheterization method in time to avoid more serious complications.

13.2.7 Urethral Stricture

The incidence of urethral stricture is about 5%, only seen in males. Although cytological analysis shows that inflammation caused by hydrophilic-coated catheters is less, whether it can reduce the incidence of urethral stricture requires more evidence. The risk of stricture formation increases over time, with most strictures appearing after 5 years. Gentle catheter insertion and the use of lubricants can reduce its incidence. Urethral stricture may be the result of repeated minor injuries causing an inflammatory response and is more common in patients self-performing CIC. Difficulty in catheter insertion may indicate the occurrence of urethral stricture. Patients with high catheterization frequency have a lower incidence of the above urethral changes, possibly because these patients are more skilled in CIC techniques, thus reducing the chance of urethral injury.

1. Prevention: Be fully familiar with the CIC process to avoid injury caused by catheterization. Research reports that the smoothness of the catheter surface is an important factor in the occurrence of urethral stricture, and the probability of urethral stricture may be reduced when using hydrophilic catheters. Therefore, hydrophilic catheters should be chosen for CIC whenever possible.
2. Treatment: If urethral stricture occurs, seek medical attention promptly. Treatment may involve the placement of a catheter in the urethra.

13.3 Bladder-Related Complications

13.3.1 Hematuria

It is normal for patients undergoing CIC treatment to have hematuria, but it should not persist. Bladder bleeding is manifested by the color of the drained urine turning red. UTI or urethral stricture can easily cause bleeding. Hematuria can also be caused by the urethra, usually with fresh blood at the urethral orifice or blood at the tip of the catheter after catheterization.

1. Prevention: The catheter should not be inserted too deep into the bladder to avoid damaging the bladder wall.
2. Treatment: Oral medication can be used for treatment.

13.3.2 Bladder Stones

Long-term CIC significantly increases the incidence of bladder stones in children and adults, especially in patients with a history of appendiceal outlet surgery. The pathogenesis is usually pubic hair above the pubis entering the bladder and becoming the core of stone formation. Mucus plays an important role in the formation of bladder stones after bladder augmentation surgery. In addition, studies have shown that the mucus calcium-phosphate ratio may be a predictive indicator of future stone formation.

1. Prevention: The catheterization movement should be gentle to avoid bringing foreign objects into the bladder.
2. Treatment: If bladder stones occur, seek medical treatment promptly. More aggressive measures should be taken to clear bladder mucus to prevent stone formation.

13.3.3 Bladder Perforation

This is a rare complication, with only sporadic reports, mostly occurring after bladder augmentation surgery or in bladders with bladder anastomosis.

1. Prevention: After bladder augmentation surgery, continuous catheterization should be performed for a sufficient length of time to ensure full healing of the bladder anastomoses. Use a soft catheter; do not insert too deep into the bladder to avoid damaging the bladder wall.
2. Treatment: The treatment method is to keep the catheter in place for continuous drainage for 7–10 days, while antibiotic treatment is given. If leakage still exists, surgical treatment (such as cystostomy) may be required.

13.3.4 Knotting of the Catheter Inside the Bladder

Knotting of the urinary catheter inside the bladder is extremely rare, often due to excessive insertion of the catheter or improper procedure. When the catheter knot cannot be removed, a flexible cystoscope can be considered for treatment.

13.4 Epididymo-orchitis

Epididymitis is common in patients undergoing CIC, with varying incidence rates reported in the literature. This infection is more common in patients with urethral stricture. Studies show a very wide range of incidence rates, from 3% to 12% in the short term and over 40% in the long term, with a sevenfold increase in risk. Epididymitis or epididymo-orchitis is also one of the most common genital infections in male patients with spinal cord injuries who self-perform CIC [20].

1. Prevention: Overall, such complications are relatively rare and do not require special prevention. Standard CIC treatment is sufficient.
2. Treatment: Patients undergoing CIC who develop epididymitis should be treated with antibiotics. The choice and duration of antibiotic use should refer to relevant guidelines.

In conclusion, there are many complications of CIC, but all of these are preventable and treatable. Incorrect procedure of CIC, insufficient fluid intake, inability to catheterize in time, and inadequate training are all factors related to CAUTI.

Nurses and doctors should provide targeted training and guidance according to the patient's specific situation, which is an important measure to prevent complications.

References

1. Igawa Y, Wyndaele JJ, Nishizawa O. Catheterization: possible complications and their prevention and treatment [J]. Int J Urol. 2008;15(6):481–5. https://doi.org/10.1111/j.1442-2042.2008.02075.x.
2. Saint S, Chenoweth CE. Biofilms and catheter-associated urinary tract infections [J]. Infect Dis Clin N Am. 2003;17(2):411–32. https://doi.org/10.1016/s0891-5520(03)00011-4.
3. Stein R, Bogaert G, Dogan HS, et al. EAU/ESPU guidelines on the management of neurogenic bladder in children and adolescent part I diagnostics and conservative treatment [J]. Neurourol Urodyn. 2020;39(1):45–57. https://doi.org/10.1002/nau.24211.
4. Moore KN, Fader M, Getliffe K. Long-term bladder management by intermittent catheterisation in adults and children [J]. Cochrane Database Syst Rev. 2007;4:CD006008. https://doi.org/10.1002/14651858.CD006008.pub2.
5. Heard L, Buhrer R. How do we prevent UTI in people who perform intermittent catheterization? [J]. Rehabil Nurs. 2005;30(2):44–5, 61. https://doi.org/10.1002/j.2048-7940.2005.tb00358.x.
6. Woodbury MG, Hayes KC, Askes HK. Intermittent catheterization practices following spinal cord injury: a national survey [J]. Can J Urol. 2008;15(3):4065–71.
7. Moy MT, Amsters D. Urinary tract infection in clients with spinal cord injury who use intermittent clean self catheterisation [J]. Aust J Adv Nurs. 2004;21(4):35–40.
8. Wyndaele JJ. Intermittent catheterization: which is the optimal technique? [J]. Spinal Cord. 2002;40(9):432–7. https://doi.org/10.1038/sj.sc.3101312.
9. Cardenas DD, Hoffman JM. Hydrophilic catheters versus noncoated catheters for reducing the incidence of urinary tract infections: a randomized controlled trial [J]. Arch Phys Med Rehabil. 2009;90(10):1668–71. https://doi.org/10.1016/j.apmr.2009.04.010.
10. Jepson RG, Williams G, Craig JC. Cranberries for preventing urinary tract infections [J]. Cochrane Database Syst Rev. 2012;10(10):CD001321. https://doi.org/10.1002/14651858.CD001321.pub5.
11. Berger CN, Crepin VF, Jepson MA, et al. The mechanisms used by enteropathogenic Escherichia coli to control filopodia dynamics [J]. Cell Microbiol. 2009;11(2):309–22. https://doi.org/10.1111/j.1462-5822.2008.01254.x.
12. Ye D, Chen Y, Jian Z, et al. Catheters for intermittent catheterization: a systematic review and network meta-analysis [J]. Spinal Cord. 2021;59(6):587–95. https://doi.org/10.1038/s41393-021-00620-w.
13. Flores-Mireles A, Hreha TN, Hunstad DA. Pathophysiology, treatment, and prevention of catheter-associated urinary tract infection [J]. Top Spinal Cord Inj Rehabil. 2019;25(3):228–40. https://doi.org/10.1310/sci2503-228.
14. Vazouras K, Velali K, Tassiou I, et al. Antibiotic treatment and antimicrobial resistance in children with urinary tract infections [J]. J Glob Antimicrob Resist. 2020;20:4–10. https://doi.org/10.1016/j.jgar.2019.06.016.
15. Naber KG, Llorens L, Kaniga K, et al. Intravenous doripenem at 500 milligrams versus levofloxacin at 250 milligrams, with an option to switch to oral therapy, for treatment of complicated lower urinary tract infection and pyelonephritis [J]. Antimicrob Agents Chemother. 2009;53(9):3782–92. https://doi.org/10.1128/aac.00837-08.
16. Fritzenwanker M, Imirzalioglu C, Herold S, et al. Treatment options for carbapenem-resistant gram-negative infections [J]. Dtsch Arztebl Int. 2018;115(20–21):345–52. https://doi.org/10.3238/arztebl.2018.0345.
17. Simões e Silva AC, Oliveira EA, Mak RH. Urinary tract infection in pediatrics: an overview [J]. J Pediatr (Rio J). 2020;96(Suppl 1):65–79. https://doi.org/10.1016/j.jped.2019.10.006.
18. Santos-Pérez De La Blanca R, Medina-Polo J, González-Padilla D, et al. Evaluation of quality of life and self-reported complications in patients with clean intermittent catheterization: an observational study [J]. J Wound Ostomy Continence Nurs. 2023;50(5):400–5. https://doi.org/10.1097/won.0000000000001002.
19. Singh R, Rohilla RK, Sangwan K, et al. Bladder management methods and urological complications in spinal cord injury patients [J]. Indian J Orthop. 2011;45(2):141–7. https://doi.org/10.4103/0019-5413.77134.
20. Ku JH, Jung TY, Lee JK, et al. Influence of bladder management on epididymo-orchitis in patients with spinal cord injury: clean intermittent catheterization is a risk factor for epididymo-orchitis [J]. Spinal Cord. 2006;44(3):165–9. https://doi.org/10.1038/sj.sc.3101825.

14 Voiding Training and Biofeedback Therapy Should Be Considered During the CIC in Children

Jian-Guo Wen

Infants and children with NB often undergo CIC due to dysuria. These patients are in a state of growth and development, and some of them will see improvements in bladder function and pelvic floor control with the increase of age. Voiding training and biofeedback therapy can help improve these patients' bladder function and pelvic floor control. The purpose of voiding training and biofeedback therapy for CIC patients is to transform those who rely entirely on CIC for urination into partial (morning and evening) CIC patients after treatment, effectively reducing the frequency of CIC sessions. It also aims to free some CIC patients from their dependence on CIC. This section will focus on the methods of voiding training and biofeedback therapy and how these methods can promote the recovery of voiding function in CIC patients. For patients with different conditions, in addition to performing CIC, they can also choose partial voiding training and pelvic floor training or voiding training combined with biofeedback therapy. These measures provide a more comprehensive diagnosis and nursing approach for CIC patients' recovery [1].

J.-G. Wen (✉)
Pediatric Urodynamic Center/Department of Urology, First Affiliated Hospital of Zhengzhou University, Zhengzhou, China

14.1 Voiding Training

14.1.1 Characteristics of Children's Voiding

Normal voiding and control functions are influenced by a series of related neurological and tissue structure factors and become complex due to their association with social environment and cognitive behavior factors.

Normal urination activity: After the development of voiding function matures, conscious activities can change the process of urine storage and voiding within a certain range, and voiding can be initiated or interrupted at will. Both the storage and voiding processes involve conscious participation: when the bladder is not full, the cerebral cortex can voluntarily relieve the inhibition of the pontine micturition center and urinate; when the urge to urinate appears, voiding can be delayed to a certain extent, and voiding can be interrupted consciously during the process. Conscious voiding is a high-level neural activity controlled by the cerebral cortex micturition center [2].

Children's voiding activity: Voiding control is a conditioned reflex gradually mastered through postnatal learning and training. Correct voiding training is beneficial for the development of voiding control. Human infants cannot control voiding because the cerebral cortex voiding control center has not fully developed, while the

J.-G. Wen (ed.), *Progress in Clean Intermittent Catheterization*, Experts' Perspectives on Medical Advances, https://doi.org/10.1007/978-981-97-5021-4_14

subcortical voiding control center is well developed, so they will unconsciously reflexively urinate [3]. For example, newborns have reflexive coordinated voiding, which does not require conscious activity participation and only needs the detrusor to contract and the urethral sphincter to relax, and the two are coordinated to excrete urine. As age increases, the nervous system continues to develop, the voiding control center and the peripheral nervous system gradually mature, the micturition control center shifts from low level to high level, and the central nerve that inhibits the contraction of the detrusor is well developed, into consciousness-controlled voiding. Normally, the bladder function, urethral function, and coordination of bladder and urethral function increasingly perfect by postnatal development and training, gradually forming conscious voiding [4].

Control normal voiding activity, even if the bladder detrusor does not contract, the bladder fills to a certain extent, and the child perceives the voiding signal and can also control voiding through increasing abdominal pressure, relaxing the urethral sphincter, and (or) relaxing the pelvic floor muscles.

14.1.2 Potty Training

Potty training refers to helping voiding or defecation in a certain posture, including legs up, buttocks down, back against the adult's abdomen, and letting the child's buttocks above the toilet or potty. At the same time, make a "shush" sound, and the child, in response, will make a "um" sound when urinating or defecating, and induce the child's voiding and defecation on this basis. Research has shown through recording neonatal EEG that bladder filling can significantly increase cortical discharge, and voiding control in infancy involves complex neural pathways and high-level neural centers. Other research shows that sphincter autonomous control is obtained at 9 months of age, which can serve as a theoretical basis for starting voiding training.

Potty training method: Generally choose about 30–40 minutes after feeding, or just waking up, using the traditional potty training method, pay attention to the comfort and security of the child's position, each time should not be too long, 1–3 minutes is appropriate, and this can be supplemented with whistle, "shush" sound, or the sound of running water to stimulate and induce voiding [5].

Indications: Voiding training can be started in infancy, and literature reports that the earliest age to start potty training is 6 months. Domestic research also shows that infants and toddlers starting potty training within 12 months after birth can effectively reduce the occurrence of abnormal voiding in childhood.

14.1.3 Behavioral Cognitive Training

Behavioral cognitive training includes toilet training and proper cognition cultivation. Toilet training refers to children who can walk practicing voiding and defecation on a toilet or squat toilet. Through such training, toddlers are trained to urinate and defecate regularly, keeping the perineum clean and dry. Family education plays a very important role in the process of children's cognition of correct voiding behavior. Parents need to have correct cognition and cultivate good living as well as eating and defecation habits for children [6].

Method: The premise of toilet training is that toddlers can walk and can independently complete actions such as sitting and standing. Choose appropriate tools, such as toilets, and regularly let children practice actions such as putting on and taking off pants, sitting on the toilet or squatting, and training toilet behavior. Children may start to show restlessness and leg clamping or express their wishes through imitation sounds or language at a certain age. At this time, they should guide behavior cognition correctly, encourage the expression of defecation intentions; guide correct defecation behavior, places, timing, and posture; and help with hygiene cleaning. The interval between voiding during the daytime is gradually prolonged, and the child remains dry after waking up, and nighttime voiding training can be carried out.

The amount of water intake should be appropriately restricted before and after dinner, urinate before going to bed, and wake up to urinate at night if necessary [7].

Indications: Usually, children can keep dry and last for several hours at the age of 1.5–2 years, and defecation is fixed at a certain time period, which indicates that they are ready to start voiding and defecation training. In addition, attention should be paid to the child's psychological and emotional preparation. When the child develops an interest in voiding and defecation and related behaviors, it means that they are psychologically and emotionally prepared. Some teams have studied the prevalence of NE and the impact of diaper usage and voiding training on enuresis, and it was concluded that children who start voiding training earlier and use fewer diapers had a lower prevalence of NE and strengthening voiding training was helpful to reduce the incidence of NE in children [8].

14.1.4 Children's Bladder Training

Bladder training or children's voiding training refers to improving the bladder storage and voiding functions through conscious control and some functional exercises. It mainly includes timed voiding, delayed voiding, reflexive (trigger point) voiding training, compensatory voiding training (Valsalva breath-holding method and Credé maneuver), pelvic floor muscle training, and anal stretch training [9].

Method

1. Timed voiding: The goal is to control bladder capacity, reduce the occurrence of urinary incontinence, and prevent damage to the upper urinary tract from high bladder pressure. Based on the recorded drinking volume, voiding frequency, and voided volume in the voiding diary, voiding activities can be regularly carried out in conjunction with the drinking plan. Children with low bladder compliance should use the safe bladder capacity from UDS as a reference for voiding volume, establish voiding interval times, and regularly follow up on bladder pressure changes to adjust voiding interval times. For children with a small safe capacity but some autonomous voiding ability, they can void for the second time a few minutes after the first voiding to minimize PVR after bladder voiding; if the bladder capacity does not increase with age or bladder contractions or ureteral reflux occur, then bladder augmentation surgery should be considered to improve bladder compliance [10].
2. Delayed voiding: Actively delay the voiding interval time to increase the perceived bladder capacity, reduce the number of voidings, and suppress overactive bladder activity. Some children may feel urgency before the onset of unstable detrusor contractions and can contract the sphincter muscle to block the occurrence of urinary incontinence, ultimately interrupting the contraction of the detrusor muscle. Children with CIC generally have low bladder function or weak bladder muscle contractions and rarely need delayed voiding training.
3. Trigger point voiding training: Before catheterization, find stimulation points to induce bladder muscle contractions, such as gently tapping the pubic area or the upper 1/3 inside of the thigh, pulling pubic hair, squeezing the clitoris (penis), or manually stimulating the anus to induce reflexive bladder contractions, resulting in voiding. Its essence is to stimulate the sacral reflex to urinate, and its premise is to have a complete sacral nerve reflex arc [11].
4. Compensatory voiding training: (1) Valsalva maneuver: During voiding, increase abdominal pressure by holding your breath, tightening your abdominal muscles, etc., to squeeze the urine out of the body. (2) Credé maneuver: It is a method to assist voiding by pressing the lower abdomen or behind the pubic bone to squeeze the bladder. You can use your fist to press 3 cm below the navel, and roll toward the pubic bone, and the movement is slow and gentle, while increasing abdominal pressure to help urinate. It can effectively improve voiding and reduce PVR.

5. Pelvic floor muscle training: By consciously repeatedly contracting and relaxing the striated muscles around the urinary and reproductive organs, including the urethral sphincter, to enhance the contraction ability of the pelvic floor muscles, such as (1) autonomously contracting the pelvic floor muscles (perineum and anal sphincter) without contracting the lower limb, abdominal and buttock muscles; each contraction lasts 5–10 seconds, each group repeats 10–20 times, 3 groups per day. (2) Do breathing exercises, contract the muscles around the anus when inhaling, maintain for 5–10 seconds, and relax when exhaling. (3) Sit on a chair, and slowly contract the pelvic floor muscles around the anus, vagina, and urethra from back to front, similar to preventing anal gas for 10 seconds, and then slowly relax. (4) Sit on the toilet, legs apart, start urinate, consciously contract the pelvic floor muscles midway to interrupt the urine flow, repeat voiding, stop voiding, and repeat many times, to enhance the strength of the pelvic floor muscles supporting the urethra, bladder, uterus, and rectum, enhance the ability to control voiding, improve urinary incontinence, inhibit overactive bladder muscles.
6. Anal stretch training: Wearing a finger cuff on the index or middle finger, applying lubricating oil, slowly inserting it into the anus, and slowly and continuously pulling the rectal wall toward the anal side can effectively alleviate spasms of the internal and external anal sphincters, while expanding the rectal cavity, inducing intestinal reflexes, and promoting fecal mass excretion. Meanwhile, the pelvic floor muscles are relaxed, and then use the Valsalva maneuver to empty the bladder.

Indications

7. Timed voiding is suitable for children with bladder sensation dysfunction, huge bladder voided capacity, severe low compliance bladder, or children with the above conditions.
8. Delayed voiding is suitable for urinary frequency, urgency, and incontinence caused by overactive detrusor or unstable detrusor, small bladder voided capacity but normal actual bladder capacity (such as normal bladder capacity after anesthesia), and children with no clear organic lower urinary tract obstruction. It is contraindicated in severe low compliance bladder and organic bladder capacity reduction, that is, those with clear organic lower urinary tract dysfunction.
9. Trigger point voiding is not a safe voiding mode, only suitable for a few patients with dysuria caused by suprasacral spinal cord lesions: detrusor-sphincter function coordination. The bladder contraction is easily triggered, and the pressure is within a safe range during contraction, and the contraction time is sufficient; there is no urinary incontinence. It is contraindicated in patients with poor detrusor contraction, inducing non-coordinated voiding, bladder pressure continuously higher than 40 cmH_2O, bladder ureteral reflux, small bladder capacity, and persistent recurrent urinary tract infection.
10. Compensatory voiding may cause bladder pressure to exceed the safe range and VUR, which can cause damage to the upper urinary tract, and it is not recommended for routine use in clinical practice. It is only suitable for patients with sacral nerve lesions who have no reflex in the detrusor and no VUR, those with weak abdominal muscle contraction, and those with poor contraction of the urethral sphincter. It is necessary to follow up by UDS and monitor the upper urinary tract safety. Contraindications mainly include the presence of VUR, BOO, DSD, hydronephrosis, pelvic organ prolapse, symptomatic urinary tract infection, hernia, etc.
11. Pelvic floor muscle training is suitable for incompletely denervated pelvic floor muscles, i.e., neurogenic urinary incontinence and neurogenic detrusor overactivity patients who still have contraction function. It should be used with caution in patients with arrhythmia or heart failure, bladder bleeding (hematuria), acute urinary tract infection, and high muscle tone.

12. Anal stretch training (indications and contraindications are the same as compensatory voiding).

14.1.5 Clinical Application

While conducting voiding training, various types of voiding diaries should also be used to assist in training [12]. This is beneficial for dynamically assessing the patient's lower urinary tract symptoms, adjusting the training plan, and following up on treatment effects. It is simple, non-invasive, and objective. CIC, as the first choice of bladder emptying treatment recommended by ICS, is widely used in clinical practice. According to EAU and ICCS guidelines, NB with voiding difficulty or severe urinary retention after birth should immediately start CIC.

For these children who start CIC and cannot undergo voiding training like normal infants and toddlers, it is difficult to establish voiding methods such as increasing abdominal pressure or relaxing the sphincter during voiding. Therefore, for such infants and toddlers, it is important to carry out potty training and toilet training.

It is clinically significant to carry out voiding training such as trying to urinate before catheterization and toilet training under the premise of upper urinary tract safety. For some older children who did not undergo voiding training in the early recovery period, it is difficult to master the correct voiding method within a certain period of time, making it difficult to achieve the goal of gradually reducing CIC times or avoiding CIC. For other such children, voiding training can promote bladder emptying, reduce PVR, lower the infection rate, protect kidney function, reduce the damage of lower urinary tract dysfunction to the body, and improve the quality of life of patients.

14.2 Biofeedback

Biofeedback, also known as biological feedback, refers to the use of instruments (usually electronic instruments) to display normal or abnormal activities within the human body through visual or auditory signals and feedback to the patient, allowing the patient to understand and grasp their own body condition and then consciously control their own psychological and physical activities and adjust their own physical functions accordingly, thereby achieving therapeutic effects. Broadly speaking, many forms can be called biofeedback, which can be achieved with special, complex equipment or with simple thermometers, scales (such as voiding diaries), etc. to adjust body functions and treating diseases.

Most lower urinary tract symptoms and functional disorders are secondary to neuromuscular diseases, and a complete medical history and physical examination are required before biofeedback training, which helps to assess the nature of the disease (acute or chronic), identify the cause (neurogenic, anatomical, surgical trauma, functional, inflammatory, or idiopathic), and formulate a training plan.

Common biofeedback instruments include electromyographic feedback instruments, skin temperature feedback instruments, skin electrical feedback instruments, electroencephalographic feedback instruments, blood pressure feedback instruments, heart rate feedback instruments, etc. and can also be combined with urodynamic analyzers and other inspection instruments to record parameter changes and guide them to achieve therapeutic effects. The combination of the biofeedback system and flowmetry allows children to observe their own flow curve and pelvic floor muscle activity curve while voiding, helping children to perceive and understand the contraction and relaxation of the detrusor and pelvic floor muscles. Here we mainly introduce the use of electromyographic biofeedback therapy for biofeedback training and electrical stimulation treatment [13].

14.2.1 Biofeedback Training

Biofeedback training (biofeedback) is a technology that extends and develops on the basis of behavioral therapy. It is a series of self-training techniques based on learning. Using modern electronic equipment, we record the information of physiological changes in the body that we usually cannot perceive, such as electromyographic activity, blood pressure, heart rate, skin electricity, and brain wave activity, etc., and then amplify it through the instrument, convert it into signals that we can perceive, which can be visual signals or auditory signals, etc., and then feedback to our consciousness through our senses. Individuals, according to the signals fed back by the body, consciously regulate and control the self-control skills of the activities of various organs within a certain range, in order to achieve therapeutic purposes [14].

Method

1. Medical history collection: including basic information, family history, past history, surgical trauma history, drug and allergy history, treatment history, other examination history, dietary habits, family education situation, etc.; different diseases can have different emphases.
2. Inform: For adults, it is important to understand the anatomy and function of the pelvic floor muscles and abdomen, understand their relationship with clinical symptoms, and realize that they are the main subject of treatment in order to achieve the best therapeutic effect. For children, depending on their age and level of communication, it is necessary to explain as simply as possible why and how to do the exercises, in order to achieve a high level of cooperation.
3. Cooperation: (1) Position selection, adults can choose a comfortable lying position, and children are recommended to choose a side-lying position, with legs bent and relaxed. This is because children often struggle to grasp the key points of exerting force during training and often exert force with their legs, abdomen, and whole body. (2) Method of exertion, independently contract the pelvic floor muscles (perineum and anal sphincter) without contracting the lower limbs, abdomen, and buttock muscles.
4. Evaluation: The evaluation process should be carried out throughout, with dynamic evaluation and adjustment of the training program as necessary. (1) Pre-treatment evaluation, select the evaluation program, and evaluate the function of the pelvic floor muscles, including the function and fatigue assessment of fast-twitch and slow-twitch muscle fibers (type I and type II muscle fibers) (Fig. 14.1). Based on the evaluation results and the condition of the disease, a training program is formulated. Most of the striated muscles in the body are composed of three motor units, one type of slow-twitch muscle fiber and two types of fast-twitch muscle fibers. The internal sphincter of the urethra is mainly composed of slow-twitch muscle fibers, while the striated muscles around the urethra are composed of all three types of muscle fibers [15]. (2) Mid-treatment evaluation, select the corresponding training program to start training, with the therapist guiding from the side, allowing the patient to learn to balance muscle activity correctly during the initial evaluation and training. For children, it is recommended to use devices with animated games and other programs for treatment to increase interest, improve cooperation, and dynamically adjust the difficulty of training, preferably transitioning from simple to difficult to prevent children from losing interest and making treatment difficult (Fig. 14.2). (3) Post-treatment evaluation, after each stage of training is completed, the patient's pelvic floor muscle function needs to be re-evaluated, including various types of muscle strength evaluation and fatigue assessment, clinical symptoms, and efficacy evaluation.

Indications

Biofeedback training is applicable for bowel and bladder dysfunction, various urinary incontinence, urinary retention, unstable bladder, pelvic pain, dysuria, fecal incontinence, constipation, and pelvic floor dysfunction after surgery and trauma.

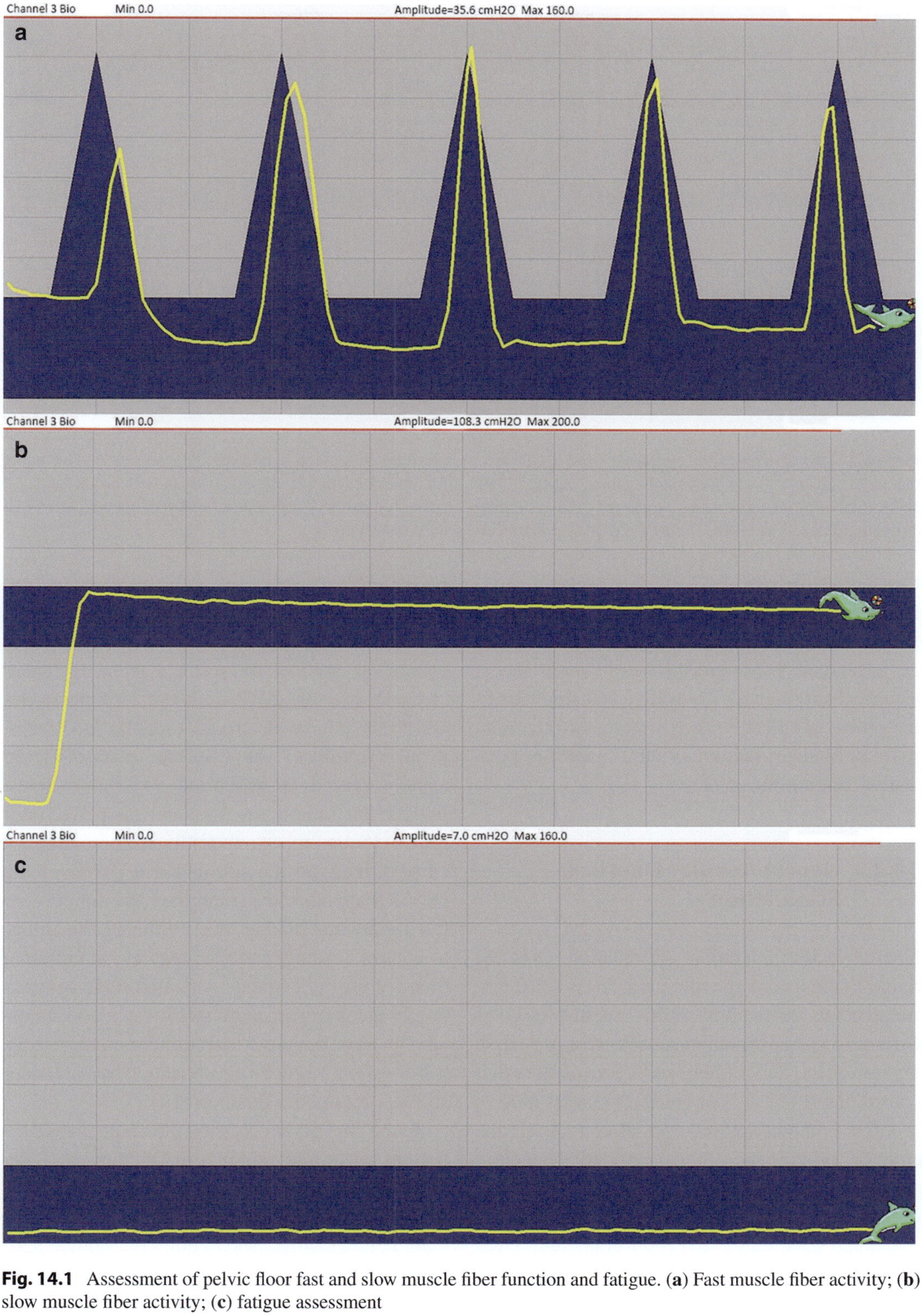

Fig. 14.1 Assessment of pelvic floor fast and slow muscle fiber function and fatigue. (**a**) Fast muscle fiber activity; (**b**) slow muscle fiber activity; (**c**) fatigue assessment

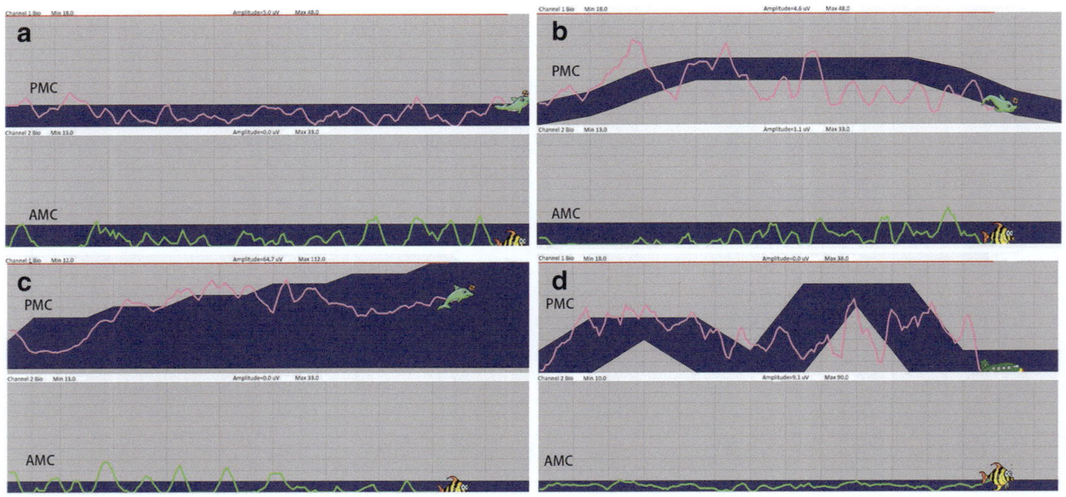

Fig. 14.2 Different biofeedback training records. PMC is the pelvic floor muscle movement curve, AMC is the abdominal muscle movement curve. (**a**) The recording curve in a relaxed state; (**b**) training record curve for pelvic floor relaxation syndrome; (**c**) training record curve for enhanced pelvic floor exercises; (**d**) training record curve for pelvic floor sensory disorder (constipation/urinary retention)

Contraindications

Biofeedback training is contraindicated for (1) those who have implanted electronic or metal devices (such as pacemakers) and cannot accept electrical stimulation; (2) those who cannot insert the probe; (3) those with symptoms of infection, such as bladder, rectum or anal infection, perianal ulceration, fever, etc.

14.2.2 Neuromuscular Electrical Stimulation

Neuromuscular electrical stimulation (NMES) refers to the use of specific parameters (different frequencies, intensities, pulse widths, etc.) of current to stimulate target muscle groups, pelvic organs, or the nerve fibers and nerve centers that control them [16, 17] or cause the target muscle group to contract and relax, or directly affect the effector, or influence the activity of the neural pathway, to achieve a therapeutic effect by changing its functional state. It can be divided into implanted electrodes and non-implanted electrodes for stimulation. Implanted electrical stimulation is generally placed at the nerve root or subcutaneously directly acting on the target organ. Rehabilitation training often uses non-implanted electrodes, which directly stimulate peripheral effectors, are easy to operate, can induce bladder sensation, and trigger voiding, thereby improving voiding symptoms and enhancing control of voiding. Non-implanted electrodes can be divided into surface electrodes and intracavitary electrodes (vaginal electrodes, rectal electrodes) [18]. Surface electrodes are usually placed at acupoints and nerve holes. Intracavitary electrodes stimulate the pelvic floor muscle group through intermittent low-frequency current, increase the strength and power of the pelvic floor muscles, strengthen the support for the urethra and bladder neck, enhance the ability to control voiding, and also regulate the afferent fibers of the pudendal nerves, inhibit the contraction of the detrusor, and improve the bladder storage function, but electrical stimulation therapy is, however, only limited to patients whose bladder still has contractile function [19].

In the past hundred years, the clinical application of electrical stimulation therapy and the understanding of neuromuscular physiology have made milestone progress. In terms of nerve stimulation, it is mainly used to quickly improve neurogenic pelvic organ dysfunction. Electrical stimulation may produce therapeutic effects through the following mechanisms: (1) simulate nerve electrical activity and control organ function; (2) block or inhibit nerve electrical activity, or enhance nerve electrical activity, and change organ function; (3) directly act on the effector (muscle), and change its contraction and relaxation state; (4) long-term, chronic stimulation changes tissue structure and function, achieving therapeutic purpose.

Preparation for children's neuromuscular electrical stimulation therapy is the same as biofeedback training, and then choose the appropriate electrical stimulation program for treatment. Paying attention to adjust the appropriate electrical stimulation intensity to the maximum tolerance is appropriate, and electrode detachment or displacement should be avoided to prevent discomfort, causing children to resist, leading to the inability to continue treatment [20].

14.2.3 Clinical Application

Biofeedback combined with electrical stimulation therapy is widely used in clinical practice. Biofeedback therapy based on voiding undoubtedly helps to improve storage and control ability [21]. Some guidelines also point out that biofeedback therapy, which guides children to correctly contract and relax the pelvic floor muscles by recording the electromyogram of the pelvic floor muscles and using image and sound signals can effectively treat detrusor-sphincter dyssynergia. Therefore, CIC patients who can cooperate with training instructions or have good compliance are suitable for voiding training and biofeedback therapy. Although biofeedback and electrical stimulation therapy cannot completely restore bladder function, they are very helpful in improving bladder motor disorders, promoting postoperative detrusor function recovery, and shortening recovery time, thereby improving and enhancing postoperative quality of life.

References

1. Narayanan SP, Bharucha AE. A practical guide to biofeedback therapy for pelvic floor disorders [J]. Curr Gastroenterol Rep. 2019;21(5):21. https://doi.org/10.1007/s11894-019-0688-3.
2. Sugaya K, Nishijima S, Miyazato M, Ogawa Y. Central nervous control of micturition and urine storage [J]. J Smooth Muscle Res. 2005;41(3):117–32. https://doi.org/10.1540/jsmr.41.117.
3. Weledji EP, Eyongeta D, Ngounou E. The anatomy of urination: what every physician should know [J]. Clin Anat. 2019;32(1):60–7. https://doi.org/10.1002/ca.23296.
4. Fowler CJ, Griffiths D, De Groat WC. The neural control of micturition [J]. Nat Rev Neurosci. 2008;9(6):453–66. https://doi.org/10.1038/nrn2401.
5. Gauldin D. Potty training [J]. J Perinat Educ. 2002;11(4):44–5. https://doi.org/10.1624/105812402x88966.
6. Zelikovsky N, Rodrigue JR, Gidycz CA, Davis MA. Cognitive behavioral and behavioral interventions help young children cope during a voiding cystourethrogram [J]. J Pediatr Psychol. 2000;25(8):535–43. https://doi.org/10.1093/jpepsy/25.8.535.
7. Baird DC, Bybel M, Kowalski AW. Toilet training: common questions and answers [J]. Am Fam Physician. 2019;100(8):468–74.
8. Vijverberg MA, Elzinga-Plomp A, Messer AP, et al. Bladder rehabilitation, the effect of a cognitive training programme on urge incontinence [J]. Eur Urol. 1997;31(1):68–72. https://doi.org/10.1159/000474421.
9. Nieuwhof-Leppink AJ, Hussong J, Chase J, et al. Definitions, indications and practice of urotherapy in children and adolescents: a standardization document of the International Children's Continence Society (ICCS) [J]. J Pediatr Urol. 2021;17(2):172–81. https://doi.org/10.1016/j.jpurol.2020.11.006.
10. Godec CJ. "Timed voiding"--a useful tool in the treatment of urinary incontinence [J]. Urology. 1984;23(1):97–100. https://doi.org/10.1016/0090-4295(84)90192-4.
11. Klarskov OP. [Training of patients with urinary incontinence] [J]. Ugeskr Laeger. 1989;151(5):290–3.
12. Jaffe JS, Ginsberg PC, Silverberg DM, Harkaway RC. The need for voiding diaries in the evaluation of men with nocturia [J]. J Am Osteopath Assoc. 2002;102(5):261–5.
13. Hite M, Curran T. Biofeedback for pelvic floor disorders [J]. Clin Colon Rectal Surg. 2021;34(1):56–61. https://doi.org/10.1055/s-0040-1714287.
14. Drzewiecki BA, Kelly PR, Marinaccio B, et al. Biofeedback training for lower urinary tract symptoms: factors affecting efficacy [J]. J Urol. 2009;182(4 Suppl):2050–5. https://doi.org/10.1016/j.juro.2009.06.003.
15. Hutch JA, Rambo ON Jr. A new theory of the anatomy of the internal urinary sphincter and the physiology of micturition. 3. Anatomy of the urethra [J]. J Urol. 1967;97(4):696–704. https://doi.org/10.1016/s0022-5347(17)63101-x.
16. Ho CH, Triolo RJ, Elias AL, et al. Functional electrical stimulation and spinal cord injury [J]. Phys Med Rehabil Clin N Am. 2014;25(3):631–54, ix. https://doi.org/10.1016/j.pmr.2014.05.001.
17. Zhang Y, Bicek AD, Wang G, Timm GW. Effects of periurethral neuromuscular electrical stimulation

on the voiding frequency in rats [J]. Int Urogynecol J. 2010;21(10):1279–84. https://doi.org/10.1007/s00192-010-1189-y.
18. Berghmans B, Hendriks E, Bernards A, et al. Electrical stimulation with non-implanted electrodes for urinary incontinence in men [J]. Cochrane Database Syst Rev. 2013;6:CD001202. https://doi.org/10.1002/14651858.CD001202.pub5.
19. Lv A, Gai T, Feng Q, et al. The therapeutic effect of neuromuscular electrical stimulation by different pulse widths for overactive bladder in elderly women: a randomized controlled study [J]. Ginekol Pol. 2022;93(8):620–8. https://doi.org/10.5603/GP.a2021.0181.
20. Xu Z, Wei H. Application and progress of sacral nerve modulation technology in the treatment of urinary dysfunction [J]. J Shandong Univ (Med Ed). 2018;56(3):29–33. [徐智慧，魏海彬. 骶神经调节技术在排尿功能障碍治疗中的应用与进展. 山东大学学报(医学版), 2018;56(3):29–33].
21. Koenig JF, Mckenna PH. Biofeedback therapy for dysfunctional voiding in children [J]. Curr Urol Rep. 2011;12(2):144–52. https://doi.org/10.1007/s11934-010-0166-9.

Publisher's Afterword

Postscript

The Science and Technology Literature Publishing House has been publishing medical books since its establishment in 1973.

Over the past 40 years, the content and form of medical books have undergone significant changes, all of which are related to the development and progress of medicine. The *Chinese Medical Clinical Masters* series has been planned since 2016, and we are grateful to more than 600 authoritative experts for their meticulous attention to each book and every detail. Nearly a hundred works have been published so far. In 2018, the series fully implemented the chief editor system for each discipline, guided by authoritative experts in each discipline. We warmly welcome the birth of each volume of the *Chinese Medical Clinical Masters* series and look forward to more scientific and standardized publishing work for the series.

In recent years, clinical medicine in China has made great strides and is beginning to make its mark in the international medical field. With the CHANCE study led by Beijing Tiantan Hospital rewriting the American guidelines for secondary prevention of cerebrovascular disease, a group of Chinese clinical experts' research results are making their way to the world. However, these authoritative clinical experts' research results are mostly first published in foreign journals and then presented in domestic journals and conferences. If they publish monographs, they are co-authored by many people, and the essence of the experts' views and results are diluted. To change this scattered presentation, as the only publishing organization under the Ministry of Science and Technology, we have a responsibility to provide a stage for Chinese clinical doctors to systematically display their clinical research results. For this reason, we planned and published this high-end medical monograph series – *Chinese Medical Clinical Masters*.

"Baijia" refers to authoritative experts in various clinical disciplines and also implies a hundred schools of thought.

Each book in the series presents the latest research results and expert views on a disease, published continuously by year, emphasizing the authority and timeliness of medical knowledge, in order to meticulously, continuously, and comprehensively display the development process of clinical medicine in our country. Compared with other medical monographs, this series of books is characterized by short publishing cycles, strong continuity, prominent themes, concise content, and a good reading experience. At the same time as the book is published, it simultaneously enters hospitals nationwide through Internet platforms such as the Wanfang Database, allowing clinical doctors and medical researchers at all levels to retrieve expert opinions through the database and quickly apply them in clinical practice.

During the process of communicating with the authors, their high recognition of the publication of the series gave us firm confidence. Academician Qiu Guixing of Peking Union Medical College Hospital said, "This project is an innovation in the publishing industry… The continuous implementation of the project can play a big role

J.-G. Wen (ed.), *Progress in Clean Intermittent Catheterization*, Experts' Perspectives on Medical Advances, https://doi.org/10.1007/978-981-97-5021-4

in promoting the development of clinical disciplines in China." Academician Sun Yinghao of the Chinese Academy of Engineering said, "I encourage our urologists to spread their innovative achievements and valuable experience to domestic colleagues, and I look forward to the publication of this series"; Professor Huo Yong of Peking University First Hospital believes that "the series is very meaningful." We thank so many clinical experts for actively participating in the writing of this series. Their hard work late into the night moves and inspires us. This is a great support for this series and an affirmation of our publishing work. We sincerely thank the authors for their support and contribution!

In today's integration of traditional media and emerging media, we are striving to create this high-end medical monograph for publication and dissemination in the Internet era, to serve the rapid transformation of clinical research results, and to serve the innovation of Chinese clinical medicine and the improvement of the diagnostic and treatment level of clinical doctors.

Science and Technology Literature Publishing House

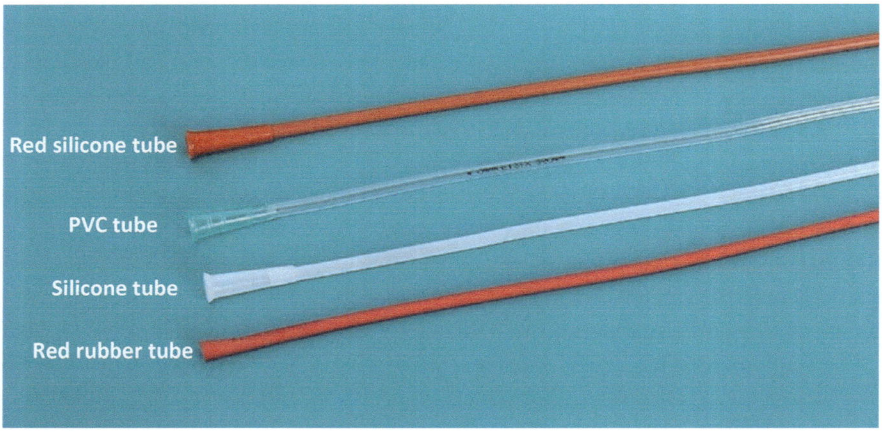

Color Insert 1 Various materials of catheters (Text page 25)

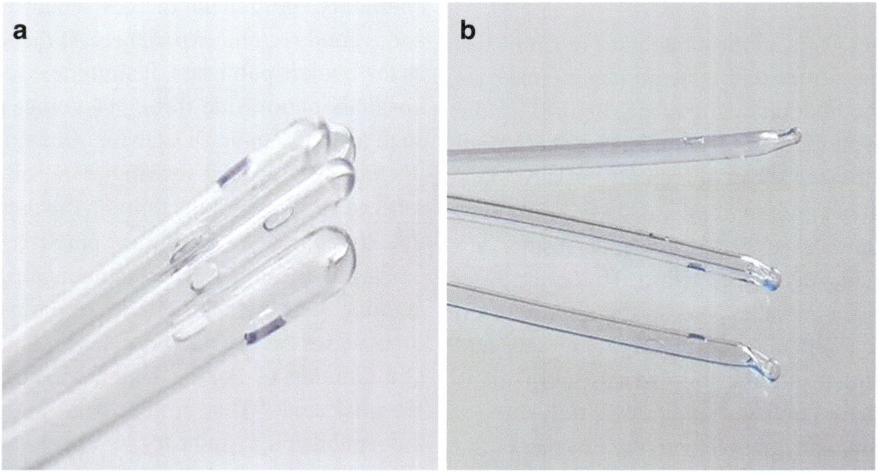

Color Insert 2 Straight head (**a**), curved head (**b**) catheters (Text page 26)

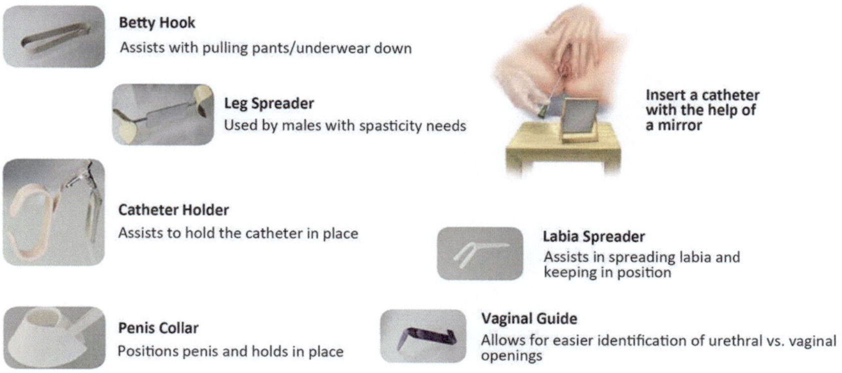

Color Insert 3 Self-adaptive CIC auxiliary device (Text page 28)

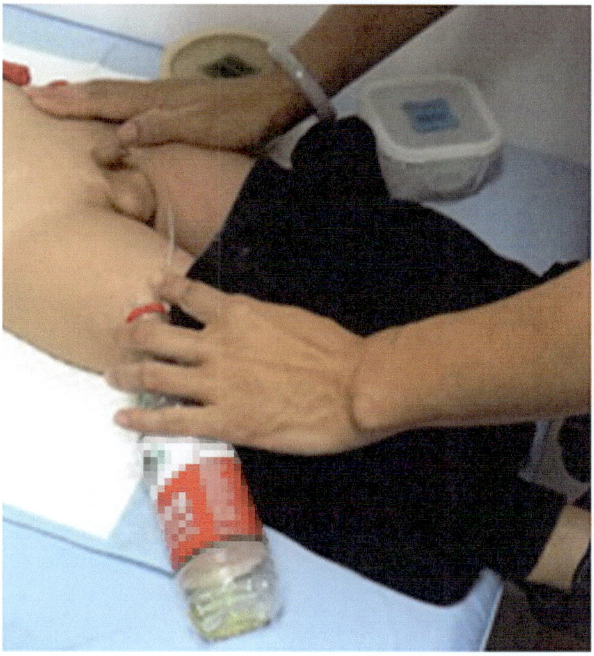

Color Insert 4 Parent assisting a 3-year-old patient with CIC, currently draining urine (Text page 66)

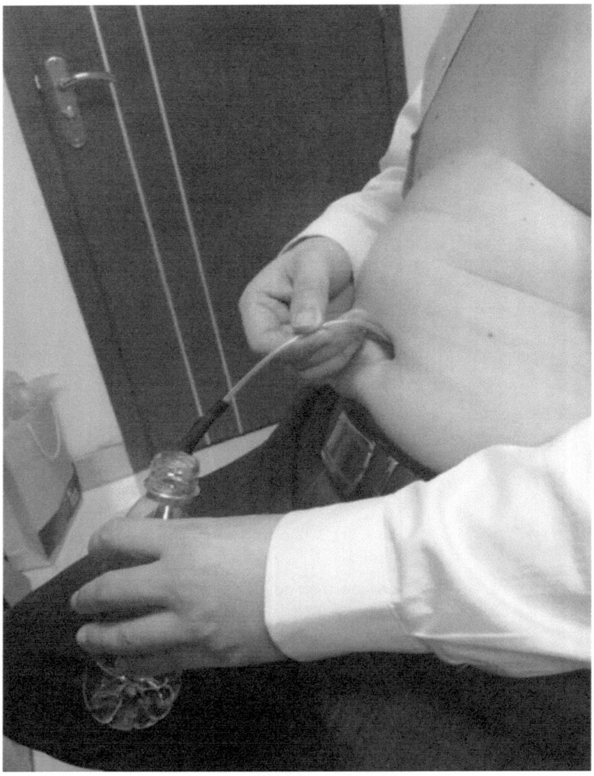

Color Insert 5 Performing CIC through the umbilical stoma after controllable urinary diversion surgery (Text page 88)

MIX
Papier aus verantwortungsvollen Quellen
Paper from responsible sources
FSC® C105338

If you have any concerns about our products,
you can contact us on
ProductSafety@springernature.com

In case Publisher is established outside the EU,
the EU authorized representative is:
Springer Nature Customer Service Center GmbH
Europaplatz 3, 69115 Heidelberg, Germany

Printed by Libri Plureos GmbH
in Hamburg, Germany